How Faith Works

Cancer Survivor

Matt Davis

Bloomington, IN 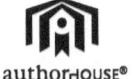 Milton Keynes, UK

authorHOUSE®

AuthorHouse™
1663 Liberty Drive, Suite 200
Bloomington, IN 47403
www.authorhouse.com
Phone: 1-800-839-8640

AuthorHouse™ UK Ltd.
500 Avebury Boulevard
Central Milton Keynes, MK9 2BE
www.authorhouse.co.uk
Phone: 08001974150

First published by AuthorHouse 10/2/2006

ISBN: 1-4259-3811-6 (sc)
ISBN: 1-4259-3810-8 (dj)

Printed in the United States of America
Bloomington, Indiana

This book is printed on acid-free paper.

About the Author

Matt Davis, the "Truck Driver from Alabama" was born at the height of the Depression on June 2, 1931, in a small community called Franklin Town, in the township of Evergreen, Alabama. Matt was born in a one-room log cabin with one window, one door, and no running water. Matt was delivered by his father's mother, Hattie Davis, a midwife. She had all the experience and necessary equipment to bring Matt safely into this world. Matt was mostly self-educated, he attended higher learning institutions and for purposes stated: "he studied Spanish I, at the University of Nevada Las Vegas (UNLV), during 1995. He entered the university under the continuing education program.

Matt was forced to leave UNLV because of his health. He was diagnosed with prostate cancer and went to the Cancer Treatment Center in Tulsa, Oklahoma. In 1996, he continued his Spanish training by taking a course at the United Way, which offered Spanish I classes. This time, he completed the course and obtained a certificate of completion. During this same time, he attended Hallie Heweston Elementary School evening classes, and further studied at Bob Stupak Community Center under a Spanish professor, where he received certificates of completion for his studies and ability to speak Spanish.

The author is an American who seeks to assert his rights to play in the American social, economic, and political system. He tells a story of his early developmental years as being riddled with traumatic ups and downs; but he has never been deterred from his passion to pursue his *God*-given purpose: making sure all children are educated. He stresses education as the key for others in a way that suggests the pursuit of it as his purpose. Matt believes that education is the key to a good life, and that it prevents shortcomings in life. This comes through loud and clear as Matt, the author, demonstrates through timelines, photos, and memorable experiences in his lifespan. For example, a famous quote of his is: *"Learn to spell entrepreneur and then become one."*

Matt has developed an educational logo program, suited for the secretary of education, to issue a national proclamation for use by all boards of education in the United States. He is the founder and director of Let's Go to School Logos, Inc. He has shown much courage in his pursuit of national approval for his educational logos, and education is the key concept. The author has made contact in writing with many if not all major politicians, and the three most recent presidents. His authority in his request for their support commanded their response, because he dared to challenge the politicians for whom he had voted, thinking that he deserved a constituent status reply and got one. During the *later* and more profound years of his life, he has been riddled with ups and downs while dealing with *cancer*, the worst of health concerns, but through many surgeries, he has used up only a few of the prayers his grandmother Mandy stored up for him.

Through it all, according to the author, he has kept the *faith*. The moral of this story is, *"I have kept the faith through my belief in God's Plan. When I get to heaven, the first face I want to see is the face of God, and the second is the face of my beloved grandma Mandy,"* he said. He thinks Grandma is going to ask, *"Matt, did you get an education?"* Matt's response to his grandma's question is, *"It is contained in this book."* He will say, *"I created educational logos for the classrooms in an effort, to enhance the education of others."*

Although living my life in America has educated me in many skills of life, I am always seeking a higher learning and planning one day to return to school at the college level.

Gods Biggest Blessings are Little Ones. Amen.

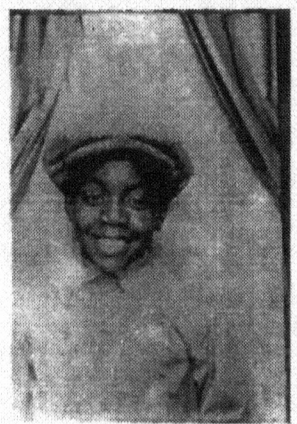

Evergreen, Alabama 1936

Education is the 🔑

Contents

Chapter 5

Chapter 6

Dedication

Dedicated to My Fellow Americans

Many politicians who have inherited the right to govern this great country of America for the last two hundred years have lost their courage to do so. In addition to losing their courage, they have lost their backbone to govern. There seems to be no interest in the one commodity which has made America great: *education for all of our children*. I have written letters to politicians to register my concerns for education for all children. In essence, my letters suggest that after all these years of doing nothing, they need help. I have taken it upon myself to put together educational logos, with the concept aimed at promoting education, that could be used throughout the United States in all boards of education. A Web site has been developed to support my mission and purpose. Please visit this site at *http://www. letsgotoschool.com*. In addition to dedicating this book to my family, I further dedicate it to all my fellow Americans, including those who received my letter in Appendix 9. See my list of politicians to which I wrote letters asking for their support of my "Let's Go to School" logos campaign and theme (Appendix 11).

Acknowledgment

First I give thanks to *God,* and then to my wife Barbara, who has been my rock and foundation for getting me through the most difficult challenges of my life — surviving my health issues. To my beloved, and friend Barbara, I appreciate you and all the things you do to keep me strong. I want to give credit and a special thanks to my ex-wife Verba, for diligently providing economic support for our four children by ensuring that all four of them obtained an education, because I was not physically there to help. Verba is an educator herself, but is now retired. However, the outcome of her dedication is evident in the accomplishments of our children. My son Terry Glenn is an attorney in Montgomery, Alabama, married to Melinda. Another son, Carl Matthews Jr., is a schoolteacher in Atlanta, Georgia, married to Betty. My third son, Kelvin Lewis, is a teacher in Atlanta, Georgia, married to Stephanie. My daughter, Deborah Lynn, a former schoolteacher, is now living in Indianapolis, Indiana, and working as an insurance executive; she is married to John Manora, who is a minister.

As I give recognition to *"God's Plan"* and ideas, positive inspiration continues in my life. I was inspired by the recognition given to me by the newspaper in Las Vegas for growing what maybe the largest zucchini squash ever seen in North Las Vegas. In the article, the newspaper showed my picture and the zucchini squash. In this article, I mentioned that my next goal was to write a book, entitled

The Truck Driver from Alabama. I had no way of knowing how *God* was going to make my dream a reality. I was expressing my desires to write this book about my life during an usher meeting at Second Baptist Church. I was passing out the award-winning flyers from the newspaper about the extra-large zucchini, when I passed a flyer to a lady named Carrie Johnson, not knowing she was in the book-editing business CJ Editing & Event Coordination, a Henderson, Nevada small business that is affiliated with Book Publishing Coordination Service. She was sitting next to another usher I have known for years at Second Baptist Church. I immediately started talking with Carrie about the business and writing my book. At this time, I give special thanks to Carrie Johnson, editing consultant, and further to Dr. Arthur J. Stovall, founder of Book Publishing Coordination Service *(www.bookpubco.net)* and the Prevention Education Counseling System (PECS) Association, Inc.

About the Book

This book is autobiographical in concept, as the author has had many experiences in life, in addition to his bouts with cancer and his subsequent survival. As the author brings his story to you in this book, his attempt is to present things in a sequence that explains them in the order of importance in his life. The author's life was riddled with ups and downs from inception, because of the absence of his father and mother, but the best thing that happened to him is that he was raised by his loving and caring grandmother, Mandy. Although many of the situations and experiences he faced existed in his life in Alabama in 1930s, they still exist in African-American families and their communities today. As a result, Matt has a keen sense of the value of education, which he learned from his grandmother Mandy, and other life experiences during the time he lived in Alabama.

His grandma Mandy taught him the importance for education, even though he first left home without finishing high school, his mother Rachel ordered him back to complete his senior year early in 1949. However, many of his survival skills were learned from his grandmother Mandy, the greatest of which was his *faith* in *God*. Matt's years as a child growing up in rural Alabama during 1930s-1950s at best was turbulent times for young African-American boys, yet he rode horses with his "white friend," "J," a kid who lived nearby at the time. Because of Matt's *faith,* taught to him by his grandmother Mandy, he was not afraid to take chances and try new things. At age nineteen Matt went to work in Pensacola, Florida. Later that same year, he bought a pretty green 1939 Chevy.

Although the life and times of Matt were emotionally distressing, he was never deterred by life decisions, and still believes it is his *faith* that has brought him through many ordeals in his life. He volunteered for the draft in 1951 for military duty to serve his country. This was at the height of a "police action"; the United States had engaged in an action to prevent the spread of communism from North Korea to South Korea. He stepped out on *faith*, as he did in many occasions, and prevailed in turning what would have toppled the average big-city kid; but Matt always turns negatives into positives, and perseveres as he gets up again and again and again. During another time in his life, he dared to step out on *faith*, and still to this day believes his dreams for his education logos will take wing. He wrote and mailed letters to many of the major politicians and the last three presidents.

He wanted support for the "Let's Go to School" theme he developed using his own money. He believed the program would have provided a boost to the economy, especially the African Americans, provided he could have succeeded in running a small business in the African-American community. Furthermore, he sent his "Let's Go to School" theme and supplies to politicians; he demanded a constituent response from these politicians and got one. He learned, on his own, how to spell *entrepreneur* and became one, as evidenced by the photo of the author standing in front of one of his properties (see Appendix 6). In addition to taking advantage of many opportunities, Matt drove a Peterbilt truck as a community servant in the Martin Luther King, Jr. Birthday Celebration. The float was built by Matt, and in the designs of the float, he includes his "Let's Go to School" logos. See photo of this float on "Dr. Martin Luther King, Jr.'s Birthday Celebration," in 1991, where Matt was driving downtown in Las Vegas, Nevada (see Appendix 8).

Matt believes that *God* really reinforced the value of the *faith* he had learned from his grandmother Mandy, especially when he had planted zucchini seeds. The seeds did nothing for two years, and then the seeds *surrendered*. One of the zucchinis grew to be the largest ever seen in Las Vegas, Nevada, and perhaps the largest anyplace in the

United States. As I thought of this zucchini, I thought of my *faith*, and the saying *"I surrender all to God the Father."*

The zucchini plant started to grow in the same year he won his fight with cancer, lower back, shoulder, and eye surgeries. Matt realized the message *God* had revealed for his future was "just stick to it." Then Matt's *faith* was tested; he had to fight cancer again and again. He knew, however, that the road map *God* had showed him through the zucchini plant would be the one to follow if he was to win this battle. Matt believes there is an enduring time in growing the zucchini; the same as *faith* takes in preparing one's life for growth and healing. According to Matt, this is the reason the zucchini plant is so important to him, and is shown on the cover of this book; it is *"God's Plan"*; you just have *faith* in "God's View of Things" and follow his plan as does a zucchini growing in life's pasture.

CHAPTER I
Introduction

God's View of Things

As a child, I spent most of my developmental years with my grandmother Mandy. Mandy was my mother Rachel's mother. Mandy and her father Jerry Franklin raised me on a farm. I was proud of my grandma Mandy for doing domestic work in order to feed the family. Grandma Mandy worked outside the home. She was paid in food items such as meat, milk, corn meal, and flour, in lieu of wages. Although I was born out of wedlock, my mother Rachel later had legitimate twins, Jessie Mae and Jesse Mack. Rachel was married to Jesse Ray, divorced him, and left the twins with Grandma Mandy.

My mother Rachel moved to New Brunswick, New Jersey, in search of work, to better provide financial support and a better life for us. My mother got herself a civil service job at Camp Kilmer, New Jersey in New Brunswick, after the refugees moved to Camp Kilmer. She later transferred to Fort Dix in Camden, New Jersey, and went to work for a hospital. She would send us money by registered mail on her paydays. My grandma Mandy could neither read nor write, but she taught me the value of life.

The mailman would sign for the registered mail for her. After signing for Grandma Mandy, the mailman would tell her to touch the pen, to make the signature legal. The reason for writing this book is because I want people to know what *faith* can do for those who believe in *God*. **"It is *faith* in *God's View of Things*** that gave my grandma the *faith* that got me this far. My grandma Mandy strongly believed in education.

I believe that if I had gotten a formal education and Grandma was still living, I could have become the president of these United States of America. That is how strongly her *faith* influences me and my *God*-given purpose that leads me to promote education for all children. I am still praying the ageless prayer Grandma prayed every Wednesday and Sunday as she woke me up to build a fire in the fireplace. I would gladly get out of my warm bed to make the fire she would use to prepare breakfast for the family every morning before she went to work. The family would kneel down on the bedside and she prayed the same prayer every time. Those words were as follows: *"My heavenly father, I thank you for another chance to pray and give thanks for your blessings, dear Lord. I ask you to come down and look over these watch walls of Zion, and see what sin and sorrow is doing with your children down here, and God I don't know how to pray, nor what to pray for. I ask you to throw your strong arms of protection around us, where no evil can harm us, and father, bless my grandson. Amen."*

After my mother left the twins, Jessie Mae and Jesse Mack, to be raised by my grandmother, she would ask *God* to bless her grandchildren. I am still praying that eternal prayer today. I wish everyone could feel a part of me, because I am a good example of what *faith* can do.

I had so many prayers stacked up before my last surgery that, if I never prayed again, I believe that was enough to carry me over. Life was a struggle at Grandmother's house for all of us, but we made it. As you read through the chapters of this book, you will understand the many trials and tribulations I have experienced in my life, and I hope you find wisdom in doing so. Through the years after I created the educational logos, many friends were very instrumental in promoting them. They used the education promotional logos in their various businesses and educational programs.

Other encouraging words came from many friends and relatives. After I received my copyright for "Let's Go to School Logos, Inc.," and created all of the educational stationery and logos, I spent thousands of dollars for the promotion of this material. I became a member of the local chamber of commerce, and the black chamber of commerce. The Latin chamber of commerce worked with me, when I opened my first store at Rancho Indoor Swap Meet, 1996-1997. I later opened a store at 913 East Charleston Boulevard in Las Vegas, Nevada, for which I had to file bankruptcy in 2000 because I owed venders $175,000 that I could not pay, due to poor sales. Also, I had to file bankruptcy because of a bad location and advertising, including all the professional people I have provided free samples to. This was a meaningful learning experience, in that I spent so much money trying to promote this idea, and nothing really came of it, but with *faith*, anything can still be developed.

A Symbol of Faith – the Zucchini Continued to Grow

Take this zucchini squash that I planted in the year 2003; nothing happened in the year 2003 or 2004. My wife and I started to grill squash of this vine in 2005, and this large one kept growing, so we waited to see how big it would get. In the meantime, I was undergoing therapy to learn how to walk again after my recent back surgery in March 2005. As times got better for me physically, the zucchini continued to grow. Then, later in 2005, the zucchini reached its full potential, ready to be picked. So this goes with my thinking that all things have a season, and *with faith and by the grace of God* can flourish.

Later, my stepson Rodney came by the house and saw the zucchini lying on the table. He said, "Pops, the size of this zucchini could be a record for zucchinis." I thought yes, maybe it could be. I took it down to the *El Mundo* Spanish newspaper. They took a picture, and then I went to Channel 3 news. I sat down in front of the building at Channel 3 with the zucchini on my lap, while trying to make contact with someone from the media. The weather was very hot, but I kept the zucchini in an ice chest in order to keep it fresh.

Finally, the weatherman came out and took it and said, "I wanted to show it on the weather forecast at 4:00 PM." Later, he called me and said, "I cannot show it at 4:00 PM, because there is not enough time. I will show it at 5 PM." At 5 PM, the weatherman kept his word and the zucchini was on the news. That is what got the ball rolling. My point is how *faith* can work if you stay with *God;* he has taught me patience. This I believe is the patience *God* wishes to instill in all of us. I had no idea this kind of exposure would come from seeds that were planted two years ago.

CHAPTER 2

Developmental Years

Growing Up in Evergreen, Alabama

My first memory of how difficult it was for my family to make a living in Evergreen was between 1935 and 1943. Starting at the tender age of four years old, I began to learn survival skills that would motivate my life achievements. I observed my grandma Mandy getting up at sunrise to go to work but not knowing what time it was, because she had no clock. She was attuned to the light and dark, and could tell the time by the sunrise, and the crowing of the rooster. At an early age, my observation skills sharpened as I learned to tell time by observing the rising and setting of the sun, and listening to other signs in nature, and later to the radio.

I knew what time my grandma was to come home from work by measuring the sunset's shadow on the ground. Furthermore, I knew the time she would come down the road. Grandma Mandy worked at the Sadies' place for food only, back in those days. At the end of her workday, Ms. Sadie would place meat and butter in her apron pockets, place a container of milk on top of her head with both hands filled with flour and meal. Grandma would begin her walk home.

After walking approximately two miles, I would meet her with a happy heart and a smile.

I would be so glad to stare down that road to see my grandmother coming. I would start running to meet her and she would be glad to see me as well. Grandma Mandy would squat down so that I could take the container of milk off her head. I would help with some of the other foodstuffs she would bring home for the family, including my great-grandfather and my brother and sister. Once Grandma Mandy was home, she would kick off her shoes, but her work was not done. She would sometimes rest for a moment, but only a few.

Grandma would start her water boiling for supper while planning the evening meal for the family. When Grandma's work schedule was long at the Sadie home, the days seemed to get longer and there was no food to eat, so I would go out into the garden and pull up young Irish potato plants, better known as white potatoes. I would rub the dirt off and eat them uncooked. They had a reddish skin, but the potatoes were good and juicy. Sometimes, when we did not have food in the house, Grandma would let me go over to Cousin Sally Ann's house. She would feed me along with her four sons, Pete, Will, Check, and Bumble Bee. Cousin Sally Ann's garden had tall collard green plants. She would send us out to pick the leaves off the collard plants. We would have to go up a hilly area and draw water from our aunt Tom's water well, because Cousin Sally Ann's well was dried out most of the time.

When it rained, there was plenty of water in the well at Cousin Sally Ann's, but when the well was low, we had to walk a mile up a hilly area to the creek to get water to wash the collard greens. After we got the water to wash the collard greens, we gathered firewood for Cousin Sally Ann's old iron stove. The old iron stove had metal pipes that extended through the roof of the kitchen. Cousin Sally Ann cooked the collard greens in a large cast iron pot. She used just the right ingredients to make the greens tender, which included Arm & Hammer baking soda. Then, to top it off, she used a cast iron skillet, to bake a thick pan of cornbread to eat with the collard greens.

Mr. Jim, a merchant, had a small store in the community where we could buy ten cents' worth of flour or meal. The flour was in a barrel, and the meal was in a fifty- or hundred-pound sack. Most of the corn meal was yellow. We could buy a nickel's worth of bologna and hog-head cheese. The best buy was a nickel's worth of bologna or a nickel's worth of cheese and a bottle of red soda water, which was red strawberry. Also, back in the day, for five cents, you could buy red strawberry, grape, Coca-Cola, or RC Cola.

When Mr. Jim would go to town for supplies, he would take his wife. If we wanted something from the store, we had to yell for Ms. Lou Cindy, Mr. Jim's mother. Ms. Lou Cindy lived a half mile down the road, and we would yell until we could see her coming. Ms. Lou Cindy would unlock the door and walk behind the counter. Ms. Lou Cindy would slap her hands on the counter and say, "Now what can I help you with?" My favorite food was a six-cent can of Pet milk and a "Stage Plank" cake with the pink icing on top.

They had three kinds of cigarettes in the store: Lucky Strike, Camel, and Chesterfield. We could buy one cigarette for one cent or a pack for twenty cents back in those days. Mr. Jim's store had one gasoline pump with a ten-gallon glass globe. You had to pump the gasoline up into the globe. The globe had numbers from one to ten. The gasoline back in those days had to be manually pumped. Gasoline was only sixteen cents per gallon, and there was only one grade. This goes to say that gas is gas. But today, gas companies have changed the label on the pump and increased the technology along with the prices.

There was a "rolling store" that came through the community once a month. Grandma Mandy had no money, but we could trade chickens for store-bought food. The "rolling store" had a chicken coop on the rear with wire to keep the chickens in, and a scale to weigh the chickens. For two weeks before the "rolling store" came, we would heavily feed the chickens with corn and bread, so they would weigh more for the sale. Just before the "rolling store" announced its presence, with the loud horn that could be heard from miles and miles up the road, we would tie the chickens' feet and secure the wings. The sound of the horn of the "rolling store" in the distance gave us enough time to get out to the main road and to meet at the store.

Healing Powers

One day, I got sick with a high fever and there was no doctor or medical facility close by that we could depend on. Grandma Mandy instructed me to gather the following materials for a "healing tea." First, she told me to go out on the farm and find some wild bluegrass that grew in our southern pastures, and pull a batch. Second, find an old gum tree that grew in the wild fields, and cut some chips off the old gum tree. Third, collect some dry cow droppings left by the cows in the pastures; we called them cow dabs and others called them cow chips. Grandma knew just what to do with all these ingredients to brew the "healing tea." Grandma would spice up these ingredients and make tea by boiling them. We had to drink it, although gagging while taking it down. The tea made me feel better and cured the fever.

Great-Grandpa Jerry the Healer

I have many good memories of Great-Grandpa Jerry; and he had his healing powers too. His claim to fame was that he was some kind of healer. People, both white and black, would drive their wagons, pickup trucks, and cars from miles around to our house for Great-Grandpa Jerry to do his work. His house was distinguished by the unique porch that extended from one end of the house to the other. It sat back off the road, surrounded by thick green vegetation that included berries of all types, a fruit orchard, big tall pine trees and big oak trees that provided shade on a hot summer day. People brought their sick children for Great-Grandpa Jerry to heal them from a disease called "thrush."

Great-Grandpa Jerry would take the child into his arms and disappear into the vines and trees that surrounded our home. The people would sit together patiently on the porch and swing their feet back and forward as they waited for Great-Grandpa Jerry to bring their child out of the wooded area where he would take them for their healing. Great-Grandpa Jerry would take a baby in his arms, lay his hands on that child, and walk across the yard into the front wooded area and disappear from view for a while, but when he would return, the child would appear healed. The parents would pay twenty-five to fifty cents, or goods such as vegetables, chickens, and other foods for his healing services. Great-Grandpa died when I was five years old. These people waiting for my great-grandpa to heal their child reminded me of my own deficits, with six fingers on each hand.

First Fascination with a Girl

At age four, I begged my grandma to let me go to school to learn my ABCs. Grandma had just gotten me my first pair of shoes. I was so proud; now I had shoes and I wanted to show off my shoes by going to primer school, as we called it back in the day; it is now referred to as preschool today. Grandma told me I had to wait until I was five years old. This broke my heart because I thought that since I had shoes, I was now old enough for school, but I loved my grandma and knew that she was right. I started school in the first grade at five years old.

I still remember how pretty I thought my teacher was, as I believe every kid thinks at that time in life; I still remember her name: Miss Hollice. The schoolhouse was a one-room building with thick curtains to separate the first, second, and third grades. They used this setup of class structure all the way through grade six. At age six, I had my first fascination with a girl; I was in love with Pearl. She had light skin and long hair.

I gave Pearl a penny, she told the teacher, and the teacher thought this was inappropriate. The teacher punished me; she instructed me to go out in the woods and break off a branch (what we called a switch). When I returned, she took the switch and instructed me to hold out my hand as she whacked me with the branch. By the way, I got the smallest branch I could find! When I got home with the teacher's note, my punishment from Grandma Mandy was even worse. Grandma Mandy made me get down on my knees and put my head between her legs, below her knees, as she whacked my butt until the branch broke up. Today, I am thankful to *God* and Grandma

Mandy for those whippings; I now know how to treat everyone with respect.

As Faith Would Have It

I was born with twelve fingers, six on each hand. As *faith* would have it, I was playing on the wood floor at my grandma Mandy's house, when I lost a finger. One of my hand's sixth fingers got caught in a crack in the floor, and as I attempted to pull it out of the crack, I pulled too hard. The finger was ripped off my hand and fell through the crack under the house. I ran out of the house and went under the house to retrieve my finger, hoping I could bring it to my grandma to fix back on my hand. When I found my finger, it was grimy with filthy dirt that had been under the house for hundreds of years; no one could fix my finger back on my hand. I was so excited and upset; my finger appeared to be jumping around on the ground and was bleeding very badly. As it turned out, I lost that finger to a bad break, based on circumstances of the times in which I lived. I was left with six fingers on one hand and five on the other, a constant reminder of the deficit I was born with.

My mother Rachel came to visit us at Grandma Mandy's house right after I lost my finger. My mother, who had lived in another town, decided to move back to Evergreen and work for a Doctor Betts to provide support for the twins and me, born out of wedlock. Dr. Betts's office was upstairs over the drugstore downtown on the main road, Highway 31. I, on the other hand, had lived with my mother's mother since birth. Later, after my mother had built up her standing, she was able to retain Dr. Betts to cut the sixth finger off my left hand, after which I said to myself: *"Now I am normal with ten fingers, five on each hand like everybody else."* Another important thing that we did just like everybody else when we reached a certain age was join the church.

"I'll Fly Away"

During my seventh or eighth year of age, I joined Sandy Grove Baptist Church as I followed in the footsteps of my grandma Mandy's teachings. I wanted to be baptized and saved by *God* the Father. I felt now I had my religion for the first time in my life. I had to wait, however for Grandma to save up enough white flour sacks to make me a gown for baptism. The white flour sacks were pure white and good for making clothes. It took what it seemed forever, but finally, Grandma had saved enough sacks and took the white flour sacks of cloth and created a gown for me. Later, on a Sunday evening, when there were at least five other people ready to be baptized, I would meet *God the Father* in that country pool of water cleared for my baptism.

Near the church, there was a pool cleared prior to the baptism in a running stream of water. The deacons would go down to this stream of running water and clear the debris from the pool. The pool was a steady stream of running water surrounded by wood, ten feet long and six feet wide and three feet deep; usually the pool was cleared before the first Sunday of any given month. The water in the pool was clear and cold. The pool was surrounded with wood flaps that the deacons would let up and down to hold and release the water.

There were wooden steps for the preacher-man and the young saints such as me to walk down into the water. Then, to be washed in the "Holy Waters" so that I will be saved and meet *God* the Father, on that great day. I was baptized in the name of the Father, Son, and the Holy Ghost and I, as a young saint, proclaimed to accept *God* as my personal savior. I was baptized in the holy waters and born again as my grandma Mandy would have said, as she and my family watched the baptism. My church, Sandy Grove Baptist, was located in Johnsonville, Alabama, near Franklin Town where I was first born.

"Now I am born again in Christ our Lord," as all the church people were gathered around the pool of water singing and mourning old hymns. My favorite song of all was "I'll Fly Away" and still to this day, I love that song. Every second Sunday in October, there would be a big meeting at Sandy Grove Baptist Church. At churches today, this big meeting is called a revival. Many churches and church people attended from all over the country. Many times, the revivals would take place the week or month after the churches did the baptisms. The churches would bring in a pastor from a nearby town to conduct the service for a week. Revivals were done to bring a spiritual awakening and unity back to the church and the people of *God*.

Our Town Had Bootleggers

Just as I was ready to pass to the tenth grade, I learned that there was more for Evergreen citizens to do than just go to church and school. There was a season in our community for bootleggers; they were called "moonshine bootleg whiskey makers." These individuals were busy making illegal alcoholic drinks for sale.

The "G-men," government agents were busy trying to catch them; they were dressed in plain clothes. The "moonshine bootleggers" caught on to the government men. They would take their money and get the size order, half pint or a pint, shake their hands, and then check the amount of money he had folded into his hand. This way the bootlegger knew where to walk and kick for the size ordered. After the bootlegger checked out the money, he would tell the buyer to "watch the kick, watch the kick," as he started a casual walk into the woods where he kicked the leaves as he walked through the woods. He kicked leaves where the bottle had been planted days before the G-men arrived in town. This way, the bootlegger never had possession of the alcohol; after all, one could not be arrested for kicking leaves. What I was learning in school, church, and the community was all part of what shaped my *faith* and survival skills.

"Hamp's Boogie-Woogie"

After sixth grade, back in those days, I attended Hanks Weather High School because it was closer to my home, but still a three-mile walk. The bus had mechanical problems most of the time, and I had to walk to school whether the weather was hot or cold and raining. "Field Day" at Hanks Weather High School was a very memorable time for me. We had exercise times once a year during this time; schools from all around the country would participate in the exercise programs; this was like having a gymnastics day like the schools have today.

My great uncle Charlie, Grandma Hattie's brother, would kill a goat and prepare before "Field Day"; he would sell goat sandwiches for five cents. During my last years at Hanks Weather High School, the principal would allow dances after school on Fridays. There was a piano in the center stage. The school officials hired a man to play the piano for the dances; they paid him three dollars per each event. His favorite two tunes were "Hamp's Boogie Woogie" and one slow blues song, "After Hours Blues." I listened attentively, standing in back of him, as he played each song.

When the man took a break to go outside, smoke, and refresh for the next session, I seized the moment, playing the same old songs he played on the piano. Also, I took the time to practice on the piano sometimes at school recess/breaks. On several occasions, when the man playing the piano did not show up, I got to play the piano in his place. I had become really good at playing those two tunes. This was another gift of *God* to me; I could play by hearing and all in the key of C. I received pay for playing at the dances, a dollar and fifty cents. This was an experience of a lifetime. Then I went on to play at the junior choir at Sandy Grove Baptist Church in Johnsonville, Alabama, where I was baptized.

Being with My Dad

Perhaps because of the out-of-wedlock issue, my dad was not much help to me, and at times attempted to make up for that. One Saturday morning when I was eleven years old, my dad informed my grandma and told me to meet a truck he was riding on at the crossroads or fork in the road. My dad was planning to take me along with the men to a town called Brewton, Alabama, to hang out with him and the other guys. After we finished the mission in Brewton, we traveled to another little town called Castleberry, Alabama, where my dad stopped with the truck for gas and I went, with my father's permission, alone into the drugstore to get an ice-cream cone. As I started walking back to the truck, two white men stepped out of the drugstore; one of them said, "Look at that nigger boy licking on that ice-cream cone." The other one, who was wearing cowboy boots, stuck his foot out and tripped me. I went down hard, but I did not lose my ice cream off the cone. Most of the men riding with my dad were sitting in the back of the truck, but did not see anything. The ones who did see what happened did nothing to assist me. I knew there would be trouble if I told my father about the incident, so I did not, for fear that the white men would do physical violence to my father's life and perhaps the other men's as well. I reasoned that my father would have been blamed for what could have become a tragic incident. This was a time when African Americans could by law be mistreated for any misdirected reason, and we had no legal protection or recourse. During many memorable events, things were distorted to me as a child.

This incident was reminiscent to the time when Grandma would take me to work with her at the Sadies' house. Mrs. Sadie, compelled by Southern tradition, did not invite me to go inside her house, but I could stay outside and play in the yard with their little grandchildren. After everyone finished eating inside the house, my grandma would come out on the back porch, call me over, and reach into her apron pocket and give me food to eat. She would return inside to work while I continued to be alone on the outside, feeling abandoned, but not by my grandmother; she loved me and I knew it.

However, I was no stranger to solitude. I lived with my grandma in an isolated country lifestyle where there were not many children my age to play with, except white kids. I had always been able to turn what appeared to be bad situations into positive and beneficial outcomes. For example, when I was tripped by the white man and I went down, but saved my ice-cream cone, this became my motto: *"You may go down hard, but you don't have to lose your ice cream off the cone."* This was very symbolic to my belief in *God's view* and *faith* that you can get up again; to *faith* be the power.

Embracing My Childhood

In 1943, at twelve years old, I embraced my childhood situation and befriended children of my own age group, even though many were white. I did what most kids in my situation would have dared to dream about: I went horseback riding with one of the white families' son. His name was J, a member of the white family who lived nearby. "J" came by my house riding the horse bareback without a saddle and asked me to climb up on the horse with him. I climbed up with his help and I held on with my arms around J's and my legs wrapped tightly fastened to the horse. I was secure, but then "J" decided to gallop the horse, which was fun for a while. As the horse galloped out of control, down the narrow path into a muddy puddle of water in the center of the pathway, "J" lost control as the water splashed up onto the horse's face.

The horse was unable to clear the puddle and fell down on his left side. "J" was more familiar with riding and was able to keep his legs free from harm, but I kept my legs wrapped around the horse as he went down. The horse landed on my left leg and the weight of the horse broke my left leg in three places. I tried to get up but, even with J's attempts to help, I was unable to get up. I lay in the filthy muddy puddle with fear. "J" said he would go for help; he jumped up on the horse's back and went for help, leaving me behind feeling alone, frightened, and in pain. As time went by, my fear intensified that "J" would not return.

I felt abandoned, as I had felt on many other occasions in my life, only this time my grandma did not know where I was. As the hours passed, I started to imagine all kinds of things like dying, feeling the pain in my leg intensify, and passing out with no one ever coming to save me. Grandma would never find me again. "J," to my surprise and pleasure, returned some three hours later with some people in a pickup truck. They got out of the truck and lifted me into the back of the truck and took me to the hospital in Andalusia, Alabama. The hospital attendants treated me with respect; they took X-rays, reset my left leg and put it in a cast, which I put up with for three months. My orientation was to always move forward with my responsibilities

15

to my younger brother and sister, regardless of personal problems that caused me to become emotionally upset. I cared for others, as I suffered my trials and tribulations of life, even to this day. I am a committed American in my church and community.

Conecuh County Training School

After I got out of school for the summer, during my junior high school years, sometimes I would go with my cousin Buddy Brown, who drove an ice truck for a small company in Brooklyn, Alabama. Buddy would pick me up to go with him to help on his ice deliveries. Back in those days, people had iceboxes or used foot tubs to keep their perishables from spoiling, and for many other uses. Most of the white families had the iceboxes; very few black families had iceboxes; most had foot tubs. The truck had a rack body made of wood. We loaded the truck and covered the ice with a thick tarp to keep the ice from melting. We would pick up the ice from an ice plant in Andalusia, Alabama. The ice was in large blocks but scored, into twenty-five-pound, fifty-pound, and hundred-pound pieces, for easier cutting; you could see the lines. We used an ice pick to chip the size for each customer.

After I completed the eleventh grade, I went to a city school, Conecuh County Training School in Evergreen, Alabama, for my senior year. There was a bus available for my senior year; no more walking to school. I graduated from Conecuh County Training School. I studied agriculture, under the direction of Professor P.A. Gray in 1950, and graduated with a class of fifty-six students. The principal of Conecuh County Training School was O. F. Fraizer.

During My Teen Years

During my teen years as I observed, learned, and experienced many things while growing up in Franklin Town, I learned how syrup was made. Grandma Mandy grew sugar cane in the fields near our home. We knew just when the sugar cane stalks were ready for cutting; the stalks grew to reach six to seven feet tall. They were taller than me and very slim. We would cut the stalks level to the ground, then load it onto a wagon, and take it to the sugar mill. At the sugar mill, they would hitch a mule to a long shaft attached to the sugar mill, the mule worked a five- or six-hour shift, walking around in the same circle; they would unhitch the tired mule and hitch up a fresh mule in order to continue the syrup-making procedure. They took the tired mule to the barn for food, water, and rest. The sugar mill was designed for the processing and manufacturing. They would stick the cane stalks into the grinder and it would crush the stalks, pressing the juice out through a filter into the tank beneath the grinder. Then they would take the tank to another area, and place it on a fire, until the syrup thickened. After the syrup cooled, for thirty minutes or so, it was placed in one-gallon buckets. The sugar mill then labeled the syrup for distribution.

Another experience during my teen years was learning to eat many foods. Probably the best of all food was pork. We had a hog-killing time, where the men would take a heavy hammer or an ax with a handle and hit the hog on the top of the head; then they would bleed the hog by using a long knife and stabbing the hog in the throat. The men built a strong stand to hold the hog; they would tie a rope around the hog's hind legs, sticking a wooden stick through the hog's hind legs. They would scald the hog with boiling water and remove the hair. The hog was cut into sections, such as the ham, legs, and head, then seasoned and dressed for smoking. The men built a fire on the ground for the pots: two large pots on the fire with boiling water. Now they would put pieces of liver and "lights" into one pot; and into the other pot hog "chittling" and "hog maws." Afterwards, the meat was hung up in a smokehouse. The smokehouse had a slow-burning fire to give it that smoked taste. They made other products from the hog, such as smoked sausage using a hand grinder, sliced ham, hog-head cheese, bacon, and pork chops.

All these memories add years of pleasure during the trials and tribulations of life. I learned to treasure each memory, as I walk with Jesus each day, and sing one of my treasured songs, "Oh How I Love Jesus." While Mom was in town working for Dr. Betts, I lived with her, and during the time she was at work, she left me in the care of Miss Crosby. Miss Crosby had a café in Evergreen, Alabama. She was a good cook; not only did I have a warm and loving babysitter, but one who could serve up good food. Miss Crosby dressed in a blue-and-grey checkered dress with an apron. One day, while at the café, Miss Crosby served me and my mother a juicy steak. I loved her cooking very much and was very excited about each meal. I started to eat the steak, placed it in my mouth, and without chewing, swallowed it whole. Suddenly, I could not breathe and I started to choke. My mom hit me in the back, propelling the steak from my windpipe onto the table. From this lesson, I learned from that day forward to chew all of my food slowly, no matter how good the food may be.

Working the Cotton Fields

During this time, Grandma Hattie, my dad's mother, was not only a midwife; she was known as a community leader. When it was time to chop the cotton, the white farmers would drive the trucks to Grandma Hattie's house and pick her up first, and she would sit in the cab of the truck with the driver. Once, I got a chance to ride in the cab, while they drove around picking up people; the back of the truck was full. I was a happy young man, although after we got unloaded, some of the young boys did not want to talk with me because I had ridden in the cab and they were jealous. I remembered this one truck was a green International with a frame-wood body; it was larger than the other trucks and could carry more cotton. Back in those days, there were men, women, and children who would work in the fields, chopping cotton. If you could carry one row of cotton, and keep up with the others as they chopped, the pay was fifty cents per day. If you could carry two rows, and keep up with the others as they chopped, the pay was seventy-five cents per day. Cotton chopping is a unique process; the seeds are removed from the cotton and dropped into the top of the hopper with a wheel attached; a horse or mule is hitched in front of the hopper, pulling the hopper down the rows as the wheels roll the seeds dropped out from the bottom into the rows.

After the cotton seeds were planted, some of the growth of the cotton plants had to be thinned out and removed to obtain new and good growth for that following season. As the years passed, I became better at picking cotton; one day I picked 206 pounds and that was a record for me. The pay was two to three cents per pound (that same year, I picked strawberries and made three cents a basket). After picking cotton and strawberries in the fields, I borrowed and rode my uncle Joseph's mule, named "Old George." Later, I saw my youngest uncle; "Good Child" was his nickname. Uncle "Good Child" rode the family mule, named "Cora." I climbed up on "Old George," then decided to ride sidesaddle. While riding sidesaddle, I had a branch from the tree used to make the mule move faster, but I decided to stick it in his ear. "Old George" dumped me on the back of my head and shoulder, knocking me breathless and putting my lights out for a while. When I woke up, my Uncle "Good Child" was shaking me with tears in his eyes. He thought I was a goner!

CHAPTER 3
Keeping the Faith

"You Don't Have to Lose Your Ice Cream"

I got a real job working for an influential family who had many acres of land. a grist mill that ground up corn and even wheat; they had a general store. I worked after school and weekends to buy food and clothes for my brother, Jesse Mack and sister, Jessie Mae. Also I was able to pick up things I wanted at the general store for Grandma. Grandma would tell me the items she wanted, which included snuff and coffee. In those days, I worked hard for the white folks, but most of the time, they gave me food items, and then at other times, they paid money for a hard day's work. After working for one year, they finally ended my employment and decided I was twenty-nine cents in debt to them. Because of my family values and *faith* instilled in me by Grandma Mandy, I did not appreciate or accept the impact of what I was going through, but it did not deter my motivation to be knocked down and hold on to my ice cream. I always remembered from experience, you may go down hard, but *"you don't have to lose your ice cream"*; and knocked down I was, but I am still eating ice cream.

Hunting with Uncle Lo D

My grandma loved to dress and cook wild animals, so I started to hunt certain animals for her; she loved to eat squirrel and skunk. The locals referred to skunks as polecats. When I could afford the shells to shoot, my Uncle Lo D would take me hunting at night. He had some dogs that would chase the animals; the skunks would sometimes spray the dogs. When an opportune time availed, my uncle and I would shoot the squirrels or skunks and take them to Grandma for the food preparation process. She knew just how to dress the meat for consumption; she would hold the skunk under water and take the appropriate nine muscles out of the skunk and presoak using hot, salty water to remove the wild taste before cooking.

These muscles had something to do with the smell of the skunk. Once, when we were on a hunt, I got sprayed. I was unable to get the scent off my clothing before school the next day, and went to school smelling like skunk spray; the teacher removed me from class. I was expelled from school for two weeks, because I had been unable to get the smell off my body, and out off my clothes prior to going to school. As I matured, I became very good at shooting firearms, especially after going hunting with my Uncle Lo D for many years.

One winter, I went over to my cousin Namp's house, where there were bunches of rice birds in the top of a tree; rice birds are like blackbirds, but they are edible. My cousin Namp had given his son a twelve-gauge shotgun with an extra-long barrel. I had one shell that fit the gun; he allowed me to load and fire the special shotgun into the treetop where the rice birds were on the branches. Amazingly, we could not believe our eyes; birds were falling out of the tree top, the wounded ones jumping around all over the place, but most of them dead. We took sticks and killed those that were still alive. With a single shot and sticks, we had killed ninety-six rice birds, more than anyone before us had done, that we knew of. We counted the birds one by one to confirm our claim. "This must have been a record breaker," everyone was saying about our bird count.

I had several good times at my cousin Namp's house. Later, I killed a record thirty-pound raccoon. We had a dog named Queen.

The dog would chase the rabbit up into the hollow of a tree. We would know that the rabbit was in the hollow because the dog kept smelling and barking. I would cut a branch from a live tree and stick it up into the hollow trunk to feel for the rabbit. Once I located the rabbit, I would twist the branch into the rabbit's hair clockwise, and pull it down with the branch, a bit at a time, while I reached up into the hollow and grabbed the rabbit's hind legs. Hunting rabbits and raccoons and shooting birds out of a tree was nothing like the challenge I was about to face.

The Depression Years

I grew up during the Depression years; and times were very bad during my growing-up years. We moved across the field to the house that my great-grandfather Jerry built, once again. Times were sad following the Depression years in my state; we could barely gather enough food to feed ourselves. We had a large cat that we could not feed. The cat would go out on its own and kill rabbits, eat the front part of the rabbit, then bring the remains and place them on our front porch at night, as if to say *eat the rest!* This happened several times during these Depression years. The railroad, when it came to town, was the only hope for work during the Depression years in Brewton, Alabama.

One year, the TR Miller Mill Company with headquarters in Brewton, Alabama came to our town to build the railroad tracks. The company dug a hole for a well and built outhouses for the men to work on the railroad. The train tracks were built all the way from Brewton, Alabama to Franklin Town. This was exciting to watch as a kid. First, they built a corral for the horses, and they brought the horses in to use for dragging the logs out of this wilderness. There were many tall pine trees for miles and miles around. Then they then built cabins for the laborers to sleep in.

Boxcars on the track were used for the kitchen. The cooks would make plenty of food, and offered some food to the kid looking on; this was my first time eating navy beans. The cooks would make a big spread on wooden tables near the tracks. Their kindness to us kids was truly a gift from *God,* because we were really hungry, and the food was good.

During that same time, Cousin Namp raised a cow, which became an asset to the family; we taught the cow to pull a plow in the field. We named the cow Lert. As you know, they don't make bridles for you to ride a cow. We made a bridle for old Lert, the cow, by using a rope. We tied a loop around Lert, making a line on the right and the left side, then brought the rope back to attach to the plow. This rope design on the cow appeared to have the same shape as a bridle for a horse. Cousin Namp's son and I built a sled with lumber. To teach the cow how to pull the sled, we cut firewood, then loaded the sled while the cow pulled forward. Treating the cow like a horse, we used the same words, "Gee" and "Ha," when directing the cow to pull the load. Also, Lert would allow us to ride her without a saddle or the bridle.

Later, my Uncle Lo D bought me a mule for $160 to cultivate the small farmland. I had to train the mule; I named him Jack. Jack was easier to train than Lert, the cow; I trained him to pull the plow in the field, and on some Saturdays, I would divide the corn from the field into sacks. I placed the sacks of corn on Jack's back and took it to the mill for grinding. One day I had an accident while riding a horse; Uncle Lo D was very disappointed, because he spent $160 on the mule and I could no longer work the fields.

CHAPTER 4
Growing Up with Faith

New Jersey to Alabama

I used to travel with my mom from New Jersey to Alabama to visit; one day, we stopped at a restaurant in Georgia. I remember walking in the front door where the waiter ran over and yelled to us. "STOP...STOP, YOU CAN'T COME IN HERE!" I told her I just wanted to get a sandwich, but she told me to go around to the back door and order in the back. I honestly did not realize where I was, and how things were different there from New Jersey and New York. People were segregated in all aspects of public life during those days. I thought about it; my money spent just like anyone else's, and I was not charged less by using the back door, but then again, to keep from causing trouble or harm to myself or my mom, we left.

On that same trip, while in Evergreen, Alabama, my hometown, I pulled into the gas station and told the attendant to "fill 'er up." I walked over to a Coca-Cola machine while the attendant was pumping the gas; I attempted to drink water from a fountain attached to the Coca-Cola machine. The gas station attendant threw the hose down, and ran over to me, saying, "You can't drink out of that fountain." I asked him, "What's wrong with it, the water that is?"

The gas station attendant told me the fountain was for white folks and then he said: "You have to get one of those empty Coke bottles and run the water in the bottle and drink it like that." I thought to myself, *Who knows who has been drinking out of those bottles!* So I stood my ground, telling the man, "Do not pump any more gas in my car." I paid for whatever he had put in the car and then I left.

A couple years later, I bought a 1951 Cadillac and went back home to Franklin Town. While there, my brother and I decided to drive around, and ended up going to Evergreen, this time to a different gas station, but the same game; things in the South were still segregated. After the attendant filled the tank up, the car would not start. I raised the hood and poured some gasoline in the carburetor from an oil can previously filled for this purpose. I told my brother Jesse Mack to start the engine. When Jesse Mack hit the ignition switch, trying to restart the car, it would not start. I was not thinking that putting gas in the carburetor would cause a problem. There was a spark from the carburetor that ignited the can of gasoline I was pouring from; the can caught on fire. As I went to throw away the can, it spilled gas on my face and on my right shoulder, which caught fire. I started to run, and that did not help, so I stopped and grabbed some dirt and rubbed it on my face and arm that were on fire. The dirt smothered the fire out and I regained my perspective. It was probably a matter of seconds or minutes, I lost track, but when I finally got back to the car, the engine was still on fire. My brother was in a state of shock, pleading for help. Then I asked three of the white men sitting outside of the gas station watching me and my car burn if they would call the fire department, please. They refused to assist me with my injury or my predicament; even with the fire right by the gas pump, they still would not call the fire department! I finally got enough dirt and rags to smother the fire. This story mirrors thousands of other social issues that existed back in the day that involved the relationship between black people and white people. Through the grace of *God* and the wisdom *God* gave with Grandma Mandy's teaching, I made it again!

The moral of this story is that it was typical of the times. After two days passed, my right arm was blistered and started to smell really bad, and I went to the hospital in Evergreen. The doctors there would not accept my Blue Cross and Blue Shield Insurance; I had to drive to Brewton, Alabama for treatment, and by that time, I was very close to blood poisoning. The doctors there had to put me inside some kind of incubator with hundreds of lights shining on my body in order to draw the poison out of my system. I stayed in the incubator for three days. After time passed and my arm healed enough, I was on the road again. After I recuperated, I returned to New Brunswick, New Jersey, and went back to work for Ford Motor Company.

Finishing High School

Many times during my high school years, we would sometimes go to a restaurant on the main drag in town, owned by whites and specializing in seafood. We could enter through the front door; but we had to walk to the back and order my food. We ordered a red snapper fish sandwich with all the trimmings. We had to eat outside or take the food home, depending on the weather.

Many times, when the weather was good, after we ate, we would go to the only theater in town, which was on the main drag. We would go through the alley on the north side of the theater to buy tickets for the movie. Then we would go upstairs, next to the projector, to view the movie; there were only black people in this part of the theater. Back in those days, the projector made as much noise as the sound from the movie speakers. It was not until years later that we came to understand why black folks were sitting in the balcony over white folks. The moral of this story is, in case of fire, the whites got out safely and first; all exit doors were on the first floor!

In 1948, I was seventeen years old, and decided to get a job driving trucks. My uncle Lo D and cousin Frank, both truck drivers, had perhaps influenced my desires to become a truck driver. I drove a dump truck for the State of Alabama for a few months. Then, later in 1949, I moved to Foley, Alabama, and learned how to cut paper wood. Later, I learned to load and haul pulpwood to the paper mill near Mobile, Alabama, where it was converted into paper. Shortly after going over to Foley, Alabama, my mom, Rachel, came down from New Jersey and ordered me back to school to finish the one year of school I had left, and get my high school diploma and in 1949, I did just that. While graduating from Conecuh County Training School, I studied agriculture under the direction of Professor P.A. Gray in 1950, and graduated with a class of fifty-six students.

Then in 1950, at nineteen years old, armed with my high school diploma in hand and with new responsibilities of helping to support my brother and sister on my mind, I moved to Pensacola, Florida, got a job, worked for one year, and saved enough money to purchase a green 1939 Chevrolet. I was about to experience a turn of events in my life that I had not been prepared for in my upbringing. One day, while driving my green 1939 Chevrolet in Pensacola, coming from work at Brock's Service Station, I was involved in a car accident. I was hit by a black preacher, who ran a red light and hit my car, totaling it. The police arrived on the scene and took the preacher's statement; he implied that I was at fault. I could not believe an outstanding man of *God* would lie; my grandma Mandy would have prayed that ageless prayer right on the spot.

My story, sad to say, did not count, since I was only passing through the town. In those days, all a local resident like the preacher had to do was just point the finger at another unknown black man, and he would go to jail. So the police took me in. They told me to get in the jail cell; the jailer's boss told the jailer to turn the key to lock position and then unlock it; locking the jail cell was their way of saying, "You have been in jail, and now you have a criminal record." When I got out of jail, I made the decision to go into the U.S. Army. There was a lot of patriotism in Pensacola, Florida, and attraction toward men in uniform.

I got caught up in the patriotic movement. Also, I thought about returning to Franklin Town, where my grandma and twin brother and sister were; they were eight years younger than me. I thought I needed to be close to help my grandma raise my younger brother and sister; but I thought going into the army would make Grandma and my brother and sister proud to see me in uniform, so I volunteered for immediate induction into the service. I could still help to support them with wages paid by the U.S. Army. When I first went into the service, I was transferred to De Funiak Springs, Florida, just east of Pensacola, Florida, to process for U.S. Army service. From De Funiak Springs, I was shipped to Fort Jackson, South Carolina, by way of Atlanta, Georgia, for basic training.

The most exciting part of all this moving around from De Funiak Springs to Atlanta and then to Fort Jackson was that I traveled by train. On the train, I had a private Pullman coach, known by some as a private stateroom. My meals were served to me in my room. When I arrived in South Carolina, I was placed in the 369th AAA Gun Battalion, an all-black U.S. Army group. From Fort Jackson, I was transferred to Fort Hancock, New Jersey, for additional basic training. At Fort Hancock, I was placed in the 466th Gun Battalion, an integrated unit with black and white Americans. During this time, the U.S. Army started to integrate the service. General Dwight D. Eisenhower, the thirty-fourth president of the United States, was in office from 1953 to 1961. President Eisenhower was commanding general and is credited with obtaining a truce in Korea.

The Korean War Years

The Korean War was fought from 1949 to 1953. The war heated up June 25, 1950, when North Koreans invaded the Republic of South Korea. The United States came to the aid of South Korea, as it was known that China was supporting North Korea. I volunteered in February 1951 for immediate induction into the United States Army. I was nineteen years old, about to turn twenty in the same year, and viewed servicing my country as a beneficial and patriotic thing to do. Besides, I thought the uniform would make me look good in the eyes of my family, in addition to being attractive to the women.

I thought the uniform would turn the heads of women, and that it would make me feel important. Little did I know about what was really going on in the war! For example, men of the 19th Infantry Regiment worked their way in the freezing cold over the snowy mountains about ten miles north of Seoul, Korea, attempting to locate the enemy lines and positions, fighting their way in the bitter cold of winds and snow. Paratroopers of the 187th Regimental Combat Team (RCT) jumped from their C-119 Aircraft in an attempt to cut off retreating enemy units south of Punsan, Korea. At the age of nineteen, the world looks different in perspective to the things that can go wrong during a war. I had this unrealistic view of war at this time. I soon learned after finishing basic training at Fort Jackson, South Carolina, and Fort Hancock, New Jersey, that this was a serious venture, one not to be taken lightly.

I realized that there was much more to serving my country than the attractiveness of a uniform, or the general commercial speech-making from those promoting the service at the recruiting agencies. From basic training, I was sent to infantry training at Camp Edward, Massachusetts. I became a private first class by the end of my first year, and was stationed at Fort Toten, New York. I was stateside, driving trucks for the motor pool, and did some driving for the post commander. In 1952, one year later, after joining the service while on leave from army duties, I was feeling the prestige of my uniform and feeling young and free; saved by the grace of *God* from being shipped to some far off, unknown country. "At least for now," I am thinking, I had escaped the real horrible reality of war and terror of all the blood and guts that go into fighting a war. For now, I did not have to use the tactics learned while in training.

While stationed at Fort Hancock, one of the assignments given to me when working for the motor pool was to drive a bus. A good army friend and I had the duty to drive to New York and pick up some women and bring them to a service club. I was also on the boxing team while stationed at Fort Hancock, training for the "Golden Gloves" boxing championship. One night in the fourth round, my opponent dimmed my lights with a hit to the head. He was from the West Indies; I often wondered if he is still somewhere in New York. After leaving Fort Hancock, I was transferred to Camp Edwards AFB, Massachusetts; then on to an area called "Flushing Meadows" in New York, where we set up temporary base camp. While there, I was directed to carry a U.S. flag in a local parade. One of my flags got hung in a tree branch as I was stepping to the band music; I was so embarrassed.

Later, while on leave, I managed to get the woman of my dreams, using my charm. Her name was Verba. She became the woman of my eyes for then. I met her at my dad, Herbert Davis Jr., and his wife, Adie Lee's house in Johnsonville, Alabama, where I went to visit while on furlough. I had a natural and fun-loving attraction for Verba. I learned from talking with Verba that she was teaching school there in Johnsonville. Verba had a room at my dad and Adie Lee's house. Verba and I hit it right off, and I agreed to meet her parents. In my 1948 Pontiac, I drove Verba to her home in China, Alabama. While visiting her home in China, we fell in love and came to a mutual agreement and set plans to get married. It was there in her hometown that she got pregnant, and after nine months, delivered my oldest son Terry Glenn.

I felt Verba was a good and honorable person to marry, because she was living with my dad and stepmother. My father and stepmother, Adie Lee, were very happy for both of us. When I returned to my assignment after two weeks' leave, I learned that I would remain stateside. I was assigned to continue in my capacity driving halftrack machine-gun tanks and trucks and equipment for the post commander in the motor pool. By the grace of *God*, I was not going to be deployed. I remained stateside driving trucks and other equipment for the post commander in the motor pool from 1951 to 1953. After I was discharged from the army on February 5, 1953, I moved to New Jersey, where Verba and I lived in the apartment. It was there in the apartment where all four of our kids were born: first son Terry Glenn. first daughter Deborah Lynn. second son Carl Matthew, Jr., and third son Kelvin Lewis. Also, I have two sons, Reginald and Gregory out of wedlock by Shirley and Ann.

Discharged from the Army

After I was discharged from the army in 1953, and during the time between 1953 and 1956, I was in New Brunswick, New Jersey. I got a job transporting bricks from Sayreville, New Jersey to various locations. I drove trucks for White Motor Freight Company. I decided it was time to move on, to get a job making more money.

I left there and drove for a trucking company, hauling bricks and other freight. Moving on from this trucking company, I drove for another company, transporting produce from New Brunswick to Wilmington, Delaware.

Interestingly enough, the company had one old 1947 Dodge truck that was a problem. One of the bosses asked me to drive it off into the Delaware River with a load of potatoes, and jump out so the truck would go down into the Delaware River; this way, the company could collect insurance. I refused to attempt such a ridiculous and dangerous trick. The company eventually bought a brand new Diamond Tractor in Chicago. They requested that I pick the truck up and drive it back to New Brunswick, where the headquarters was located. This was one of the worst rides I had ever experienced. With no trailer on the back to hold the weight in place, the truck was bouncing all over the road. I had to reduce the air in the tires to stabilize the truck's balance.

I started transporting potatoes from Massachusetts to Augusta, Georgia, where I would unload them. Then I would travel to Hasting, Florida, and pick up another load of potatoes to bring back to New York. Prior to exhausting this opportunity, I moved on to another employer, a fuel oil company and drove for them transporting fuel oil in tankers to Pennsylvania and New Jersey. I enjoyed working for this fuel oil company, but in spite of all the experience gained, I was terminated for providing false information on my application regarding a back injury. When I worked for a building material companym there was an accident that caused the injury to my back; I failed to put it on the application.

One day, I was involved in an accident where a flatbed truck backed up into a boxcar on the railroad track; the engineer backed the train boxcar into a string of boxcars to connect at the same time I was unloading some insulation from another boxcar. When this string of boxcars hit the boxcar I was working in, the force of the impact caused me to lose my balance and fall down hard to the floor, resulting in my back injury. *This time I may have lost a little of my ice cream, but I held on to the cone.* After a few visits to the doctor, I contacted an attorney to represent me. A few days after an attorney was involved, the headlines in the newspaper read "MATTHEW DAVIS SUES RAILROAD COMPANY FOR 100,000 DOLLARS." After a year passed, and in between being unemployed a few times, the company settled out of court for 6,000 dollars. However, during that year, the attorney loaned me money.

After settlement of the lawsuit, this did not leave me much money. I had enough to attend a school in New York, called B.C.A. Radio Broadcast Caching Association. I received a second-class license, which led me to El Centro, California, but in order to get to California, I had to pawn my overcoat and gun in El Paso, Texas. I had overspent and partied too much by way of New Orleans, Louisiana, on the way to California. Once I made it to California, I found myself in the middle of a watermelon field while listening to an FM radio station, but I kept going until I reached Riverside, California. I left my family in China, Alabama, with my wife's mother, Eula Reed. Eula was a beautiful and sweet lady. It is not every day that one can say the mother-in-law is supporting the son-in-law. This had to be another blessing from *God*.

Soon after reaching California, I left my mom in Franklin Town with Grandma Mandy. My grandma Mandy was sick when I left her in Franklin Town. She passed from this earthly world the following February, 1960, which dealt a devastating blow to me, because I was financially unable to attend her funeral. When I received the news that she had passed, I still cannot describe my feelings, because I could not afford to go to her funeral; Grandma Mandy was my first love. She could not read or write, but she taught me the values of life, my *faith* in *God's View* of things. I am instilled with the values of life and *faith* Grandma Mandy taught me to this day. I have many fond memories of my grandma; her telling the time by the sound of the rooster and the position of the sun, and that ageless prayer ringing in my mind and soul.

While at home this time, Mom met a man, Willie D. Rogers. He owned a Bar-B-Q Pit in Evergreen, Alabama. He was a beautiful man, kind and gentle in every way as a stepfather. He was the founder of Willie D. Rogers' Bar-B-Q Pit. After a few years passed, they were married happily for many years before he died. My mom tried desperately to keep the business going, but just could not make things go. Barbara and I use to help work the Pit when we went on vacation. Mom suffered from Alzheimer's disease; Mom and my stepfather are both buried at the same cemetery near the house at Second Baptist Church in Evergreen, Alabama.

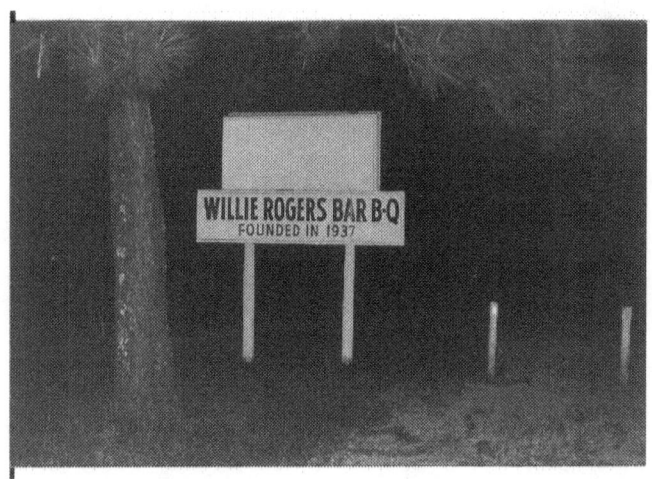

Picture Of Willie D. Rogers Barbeque Pit Sign

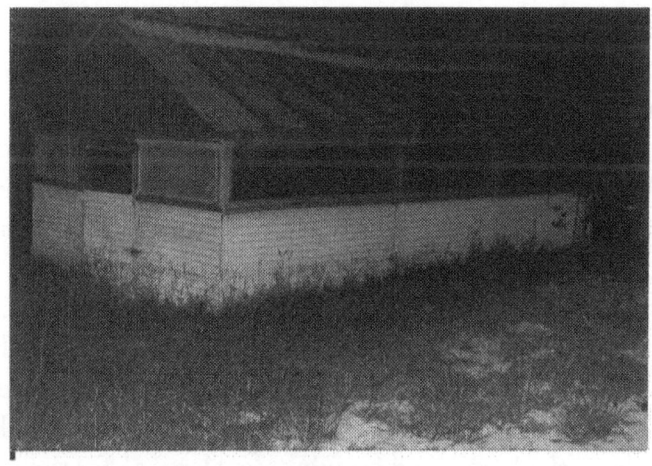

Picture Of Willie D. Rogers Barbeque Pit

CHAPTER 5
Faith at Work with Trials and Tribulations

The Street Gambler in California

I was visiting Hollywood Park Racetrack in Los Angeles, quite frequently in 1963. One day, I picked a horse in the first race, and first part of the daily double. The horse's name was Black Pool 8. The second half I picked a horse named Come Fly With Me #1; they both won the daily double, and paid $1,060. It was at the racetrack that I met Barbara a week later, after my big win. Barbara's dad had dropped her and a friend named Fay off at the racetrack. They were standing next to me, when we started talking about the horses that looked good, and picked a winning horse. We continued to mix conversation about the racetrack horses and later about other events and things we liked. About the third or fourth race, I gave Barbara a twenty-dollar bill, and asked her to bet some horses for me; I told her to place a bet for herself, but she did not. Barbara and I talked and laughed about the horses and jumping up, clapping for the horses in the races that I won bets on. We hit it off really well and we started to share our personal thoughts.

At the end of the day, both women needed a ride home. I had recently bought a 1959 Pontiac, and it was in the dealership garage and I had a loaner car, which I asked Barbara to drive. Barbara drove and dropped off her friend Fay. I then asked her to drive me to my favorite gambling joint, a local friend's house. This was Friday night; Barbara and I partied together and had fun all night. But after that night, I did not call her until a week later. The following Monday, I went to work; my workplace was within walking distance of my home. After about four or five days, Barbara came down to my job, and the two of us worked out a relationship arrangement. She had three sons: Lynn, Danny, and Rodney. After years of getting to know each other, I got married to Barbara.

Mid-Sixties Gambling Episodes

During my street gambling episodes, every Friday or Saturday, I got into fights often. Every time I got into an argument or a fight, I would call and tell Barbara to bring my gun. She would always honor my request. This kind of thing became a habit, but by the time she got there, all the players had scattered. One night I got into a fight with a man, and I had his head under my left arm while beating his head with my right fist. The man bit me, and it took a long time for that bite to heal; it was because he had blue gums. They say that if someone with blue gums disease bites you, it is poison.

Another night, I got into a fight over a five-dollar bet while gambling at a house. The man ran out of the house on Central Avenue in Los Angeles, after I was able to break away from the people holding me back from fighting. I chased the man and caught up with him, just as he was opening the trunk of his car, probably to get a weapon out to use on me. I said to him, "Whatcha got in there?" The man jumped into his car, obviously not having enough time to secure the weapon. I jumped into my car and began chasing him again for about three blocks when the man stopped and attempted to get in the trunk again. But I was too close, so the chase continued for about a mile, with both of us running through red lights. I finally stopped and called off the chase; it dawned on me, this was dangerous, and it was not worth giving my life over five dollars.

Meeting Celebrities

After this major altercation with gambling, I decided to stop the street gambling. I got a job working with the William J. Burns Detective Agency as a security guard. During the mid-sixties, I worked part time for Burns Detective Agency in Los Angeles, as a security guard. I had the occasion to meet several big-name entertainers performing at a location I was assigned to, and became responsible for the security of these celebrities. On one such occasion, Channel 9 TV was taping a show, and I was assigned as their security guard for this activity. It was a Friday night, and the stars were Otis Redding and Sonny and Cher Bono. This was an exciting time to see these stars up close and personal.

During that time, I was a smoker. My brand was Winston and so was Otis Redding's, I learned as the show progressed. I shared cigarettes with Otis during the taping of the show. Otis was wearing tight pants with bell bottoms and one small pocket, the style of the times during the sixties. Having the opportunity to speak to a man like Otis Redding was a pleasure. Otis was born to a Baptist minister in Dawson, Georgia, which explains his musical influence. He became well-known in the sixties when he sang at the Grand Duke Club, after his exposure in the church choir.

I learned that later Otis joined the Johnny Jenkins and the Pine Toppers. He sang at "teenage party" shows sponsored by the King Bee, Hamp Swain, a local celebrity disc jockey, and initially Saturday mornings at the Roxy Theater, and later at the Douglas Theatre in Macon, Georgia. As a performer for many years, Otis appeared throughout the United States, Canada, Europe, and the Caribbean. He became famous and well-known to the music industry. I considered my meeting Otis Redding another blessing in my life. To see and meet a man who has accomplished so much in such a short time was an omen to what one might realize. Later, there was a plane crash as Otis Redding and his group was last leaving Atlanta,

Georgia, on his private twin-engine Beechcraft plane that went down into Lake Monona in Madison, Wisconsin; on that memorable day, December 10, 1967, that claimed his life and those of others in his path. Strange as it may seem, Otis's trumpet player was left behind in Atlanta. By incidence, I had the opportunity to meet him while visiting in Los Angeles in 2004.

Later, during the same occasion of the show tapings, I had the good fortune to meet Sonny and Cher Bono, while employed at Burns Detective Agency in Los Angeles, during the Channel 9 TV show taping. Also, Sonny and Cher were dressed pretty much in the stylish gear of the 1960s. Sonny and Cher got their great spot on the *The Merv Griffin Show* that convinced CBS programming head, Fred Silverman, that Sonny and Cher, two of the top touring acts of the sixties, could be the network's next big thing. While at Channel 9 TV, the crowd was cheering, and became a bit radical as I was escorting Sonny and Cher out of the studio. The crowd escalated into a mob and things got pretty bad, so I picked Cher up and placed her into the back seat of the limousine where Sonny Bono had deposited himself. Many years later, I watched them on television shows and comedy hours, including their appearances on the *Sonny and Cher Comedy Hour* that debuted on CBS. Later to my surprise, and that of the world, Sonny Bono was killed in a skiing accident at Heavenly Ski Resort in South Lake Tahoe, California, on the California-Nevada state line on January 6, 1998.

Flying Airplanes

I took airplane flying lessons at El Segundo Airport in Los Angeles, and became content with flying. I obtained a license and started flying this small aircraft in 1978-83. This became a hobby I enjoyed, especially when flying from El Segundo Airport to Orange County Airport, which is now known as John Wayne Orange County Airport. My greatest thrill was to turn on the electric fuel pump for safety, and get down close to the Pacific Ocean waters, and wave at the nude people on the private beach area at the Palace Verde Cove. My greatest scare and heart-wrenching event was one day while training over the Pacific Ocean, climbing up to stall the engine. I waited too late to push the stick forward and we were falling fast. So there we were trying to restart the engine in midair, and we were losing altitude and getting closer to the Pacific Ocean, the water seemed to be coming up at us fast. We panicked, but regained control at last I thought by the grace of *God*, saved again; the engine started in the nick of time. For this occasion, I thought how blessed I had been over the years of my life escaping once again to walk a little closer with Jesus. I later wrote a song (not yet recorded), titled, "I Want to Walk Just Like Jesus Every Day." I continued to fly after moving to Las Vegas, but eventually things just got too expensive. Now if I can pass the physical, I am going to resume flying again.

The Enterpriser

The late 1970s were at hand, and this was my time to become an entrepreneur. I was in business during these years. I opened a bar and restaurant in Los Angeles, on Central Avenue at 18th Street, called Matt's Place. I had obtained a beer and wine license for the place. But in order for me to protect my individual investment, I needed more operating capital, if I was to keep the business going and recoup my original investment. In order to meet this goal, it was necessary for me to work a full-time job to keep my business operational at the bar and restaurant. Therefore, I got a full-time job working for an outdoor advertising company. Later, the company moved to Texas. Then I went to work for a meat company in Vernon, California, and at the same time I operated my bar and restaurant. I started another business on the weekends.

I converted a school bus to a party bus and started trips to Las Vegas. Another venture I undertook was getting into the music business. I formed my own music group, named Matt's Madness, and managed another group called RTD. I took them on a tour to Hobbes, New Mexico, Phoenix, and then to Tyler, Texas. They were touring with Chick Willis, and ended up in Las Vegas, playing one weekend set at Towns Tavern on Jackson Street. Later in Los Angeles, I booked Big Joe Turner, Pee Wee Craton, Hoppie Hopkins,

Blues Boy Wells, Smoky Wilson, and many more at the Chandelier Social Club on 91ˢᵗ and Mae Avenue in 1979.

The Chandelier Social Club was owned and operated by Willie and Corrine Swenney. I still have the newspaper clipping from the shows. Eventually, I closed out on the lease on Matt's Place in 1977, after shoulder surgery. I sold the party bus in 1983, wrapping up all my ventures in California. Barbara and I moved to Las Vegas in 1984, where I purchased and became owner and operator of a tractor and end-dump trailer. When I got to Las Vegas, the first job I got using my newly acquired equipment was working with a brother who was slow in payment, and later stopped my paychecks; I had to sue this brother. However, I was forced to park my equipment and go back to Los Angeles to borrow $700 plus retainer fee from a friend.

Then, I pursued more work as a member of the Teamsters Union organization. I went to work at the Nevada Test Site for a company named RECO. Later, I decided to leave Nevada Test Site and go owner/operator again. I bought a tractor from some friends, rented a trailer and borrowed four tires from another friend. After a few paychecks, I bought a new set of rubber tires and returned the four tires. Then I returned the tractor-trailer to the original owner because money was coming in slowly. I finally secured a job working for a black-owned trucking company, and this paid off all my expenses, because they helped keep some meat and potatoes on the table by allowing salary advances. Barbara and I lived in a one-bedroom kitchenette in the Linda Manor Apartment Buildings on Main Street in Las Vegas. Things got a bit rough, and I had to pawn some musical equipment that I had acquired in California. I managed to pawn the equipment for a measly $130 to a friend.

In 1986, while working on a pipeline for this trucking company on Oakey and Decatur Boulevard in Las Vegas, I dumped my load and was pulling out to the main street, which was Oakey, when I heard a voice on the CB radio say, "Let it down, Matt, let it down, let it down," so I stopped immediately. The voice I heard was that of a friend, another truck driver. I was about five feet away from being toasted by the electrical wires above me. I would have torn down the electrical power lines above and they would have made toast out of me. My friend, to this day, doesn't know how many times I have thanked him for alerting me to that potential deadly danger. My main thanks go to *God* for placing him in that position to save me. Again I thought *"saved by the grace of God!"*

"Let's Go to School" Logos: Education Is the Key

In 1994, I was driving a water truck for a paving company. I was laid off and decided to retire and get my "Let's Go to School" stationery on track. A friend made a $1,500 investment in the "Let's Go to School" project. During this period, I created the educational logos by taking the word *key* out and putting the symbol, a skeleton of a key in place of the word *key* for the Let's Go to School logos. This transmitted into my saying "Education is the Key." One of the logos is engraved in the sidewalk at West Oakey Facility of the Opportunity Village. Samples of the "Let's Go to School" stationery were sent to every state education agency in the United States. I was very proud of my accomplishment and wanted to get the words out there. My logos sounded influential and were very important to me. Most of the individuals responded with congratulations.

I knocked on many doors through the years, trying to get acceptance of the "Let's Go to School" stationery. The logos were created to encourage education and to be used as a tool in the classroom, as well as a slogan supporting the idea of going to school to be educated. I met with opposition during these years of promoting my logos, but this did not deter me from continuing my *God*-given mission: promoting education. I had some educators adopt and use the logos. There were others who looked down their noses at me, because they felt that I had no formal education, from my approach at presentation of the logos and slogan. For example, I took time off work and made an appointment with a professor at a local college. This professor looked at my draft of the logos and advised me to take it to a McDonald's in Watts, California, and maybe they could help me.

I applaud those who do have a formal education. However, I feel that it is not right for others to look down their nose on persons who do not have an education. This is why I urge all youth and senior citizens to get an education and go back to school and get a degree in something. It is practically free for senior citizens to go to school. I am seventy-four years young, and I plan to go back. I had enrolled for a fall semester several years ago at the Community College of Southern Nevada, and I was unable to attend because of illness. With positive thinking and with the grace of *God*, I feel my health is continuing to improve as I will keep on in the pursuit of education with every gust in my body. However, I too know that education comes in many forms as we walk through this life, and not just from school.

CHAPTER 6
A Test of Faith

Diagnosed with Prostate Cancer

I was first diagnosed with prostate cancer in 1995, while attending Spanish I class at UNLV under the Continued Education Program, and this was shortly after I started to work on the education logos as well. The urologist used modern technology to make the diagnosis; the doctors used high-tech cameras to gather information and analyze symptoms. Lesions were discovered in my prostate gland. During an office visit, my doctor requested his nurse to get the other doctor in his office, as he wanted another opinion; he said, "I want him to see this." The doctor continued to review the lesions while the other doctor in his office was en route. When the other doctor arrived, my doctor said: "No use. I just broke the scope of the camera off."

The doctor worked for about thirty minutes in order to remove the scope of the camera out of my penis. This was a very uncomfortable and painful process for me. During this period of time, it seemed like forever, to the point where I started to think of an extra surgery just to remove the scope of the camera out. It was finally removed. The attending doctor then asked me to bring my wife into the room, so that the surgical procedure could be explained to her. I called for my wife, Barbara, who was sitting in the waiting room. We took a seat in the doctor's office while he proceeded to explain the surgical procedure, and potential side effects as the reason for having the surgery, using a diagram on the wall and medical terminology.

The doctor explained this would be a bloody procedure. He told me to come in and they would start saving my blood for surgery. I needed to give several pints of blood to insure my safety, in case I needed blood during and/or after the surgery. The medical team explained to me that after the Lupron shot and the surgery, I would never be able to have sex again. I thought, if this saved my life, I could do without the sex, maybe! My wife and I went to a cancer blood specialist, Dr. H. J. Parks, for an opinion. I followed all of the rules for the testing leading up to the surgery. I immediately started researching the Internet and telephone directories for cancer centers; I used my computer and got on the telephone; finally, I discovered the Tulsa, Oklahoma Cancer Treatment Center. I made the necessary arrangements with my insurance companies. I learned from my research that this was a very good cancer treatment center. The cancer treatment center asked me to bring my wife along. We made our flight arrangements; Barbara and I took off that week.

When Barbara and I arrived at the baggage claim, there was a limousine driver holding a sign with my name on it. I could not believe it was for me, and as I was getting closer, the driver finally walked toward me too, and asked if I was going to the cancer treatment center; I said yes. The driver confirmed my name. Then we drove to the cancer treatment center. They had room accommodations at the facility at reasonable rates for me and my wife. This procedure took about three days, and we were on our way back to Las Vegas for a short stay at home before returning for further treatment.

After preparations were made, I returned to the Tulsa, Oklahoma Cancer Treatment Center and Hospital, where they planted 108 radiation seeds into my prostate gland. I only lost four seeds, during this time while straining upon urination, during the first week after the surgical procedure. My PSA level dropped down from 11.9 to 3.5. I could tell that all my prayers, and those of others praying for me, were working and that the *faith* of a "mustard seed" was all the *faith* I needed. I was a very happy man, and a blessed one too. After several years passed, I started to have difficulty in urination again, and my PSA level elevated.

I returned to the Tulsa, Oklahoma Cancer Treatment Center for a long thirty-day stay, in order to take radiation treatments twice per day. My daughter, Deborah, and my second son, Carl, and my brother, Jesse Mack visited me in Tulsa. I returned home to Las Vegas again. I knew that my prayers were answered and there were many people praying for me. I began going to my cancer blood specialist in Las Vegas every three months, and my progress reports were improving. So many times now in my life, I have faced diversity with my health; I have gone through so many surgeries and life-threatening situations. Each time I remembered that ageless prayer Grandma prayed. I thought of her and how she appeared to pray with a sincere heart; I thought too of praying with a sincere heart and how it can see you through; that *God has a plan* for all of us.

A Man of God Through the Years

Life has plotted a route for me through so many health battles since joining the church of my choice back in 1986: the Second Baptist Church of Las Vegas, known as "The Miracle on Madison Avenue." I joined the Second Baptist Church usher board that same year and attended usher training at Greater New Jerusalem Church. I found that I could be an usher and not have to make all the meetings. The ushers met twice a month instead of every week.

I started working with the senior usher ministry at Second Baptist Church and enjoy it to this day. I do not know exactly how miracles work, but I do know there are some beautiful things happening to me through the years. The years of my life have been passing and I wavered, but I have kept the *faith* of a "mustard seed," and now I am now a "Man of God." So many trials and tribulations, but *God* brought me through; for example, there was a time in my life I could not walk without assistance, but I can now by the grace of *God* and all those prayers. Foremost in prayers are those Grandma prayed over the years and stored up for me. Second Baptist Church is where the stack grew higher, in addition to my family's prayers, and the prayers were mercifully granted.

Also, I participated in the "Brotherhood Ministry" and I joined the male gospel choir at Second Baptist Church, the next year after joining the church in 1987. The support shown to me through the major crisis in my life has strengthened my belief in *God*. I sang in the gospel choir until I started working for the *Stratosphere*. Because of my work assignment, I could not make the once-a-week rehearsal that was a requirement of the male gospel choir, but I knew that I would always remain close to *God* first and in Second Baptist Church ministry.

During my work shift, I found an expensive bracelet, which I turned in to security at the *Stratosphere*. They returned it to the original owner, who was visiting in the showroom. I received a twenty-dollar reward for being honest. There was a write-up in the *Stratosphere* newspaper giving recognition to me for returning the bracelet. After I had to give up my service in the male gospel choir, I felt a void. Later, I could not make all the meetings required by the male gospel choir.

Eye Surgery

I started to have problems with my left eye in 1996, so I went to my optometrist in Las Vegas. The optometrist gave me a thorough examination and referred me to another specialist because of the condition of the retina in my eye. I remembered that this was a Thanksgiving holiday weekend; the doctor told me to call him at his home if things got worse over the Thanksgiving holiday. My retina condition got worse on Thanksgiving Day, and I called the doctor at his home. I explained my problem to my doctor; he said to me: "I am in the middle of cooking Thanksgiving dinner, but I will stop and meet you at my office." So I met him at the office, and he gave me some temporary treatment, and made a referral for me to meet with a specialist the following day.

After the examination with the specialist, I found that the retina had fallen apart in my left eye and I would have to go in for surgery on my eye; because my retina was detached, it would require a buckle to hold the retina in place. The doctor made the arrangement with Sunrise Hospital in Las Vegas to do the surgery. He then immediately notified me of the arrangement and explained, in great detail, the surgical procedures to me. I was ordered not to eat any food for twenty-four hours prior to the surgery and could only drink water four hours prior. Right after the surgery, I woke up and there were numerous people in the room.

They were discussing food for lunch, and I said to them in a deep voice, "I am so hungry, how dare you folks talk about food with me starving." A nurse replied, "Quiet down, you are supposed to be asleep." I was still somewhat out of it from the surgery, and fell in and out of sleep. When I woke up, another miracle: My left eye was saved, I could see. My experience with the surgery was very painful. I envisioned my eye was lying on the table and I could see the doctor's fingers turning my eyeball while putting the buckle on. The anesthesiologist told me that only a certain amount of pain medicine could be given to me, so the doctor told him that the surgery had gone over the time and I begged, "Please put me back to sleep with more medication," and they did. Thank *God* today the buckle is still intact and my vision is good.

Look What Faith Has Done

Later, a friend of mine agreed to partnership with me in opening my second store in the year 1998 at 913 East Charleston Boulevard in Las Vegas. Although there were more triumphs and tribulations to come, I was determined to keep reaching for success. I had closed the business due to illnesses, but after several years passed, I came out of retirement in 2000 and started to work again, driving for a paving company.

Later, during this same time, my family doctor discovered I had a mass in my left lung. He arranged for a biopsy of the mass in my left lung; they went through my chest. The lung specialist performing the procedure immediately wanted to remove the mass, but I wanted to get a second opinion. Again I called the Cancer Treatment Center in Tulsa, Oklahoma and talked with a specialist. I was instructed to come back to the Cancer Treatment Center for an evaluation. I immediately made airplane reservations for me and Barbara. When I arrived, they scheduled the necessary test. After all the tests and evaluations were completed, they confirmed that the mass in my left lung needed to be removed. I was given the choice of having the procedure in Tulsa or returning to Las Vegas.

They recommended a team of surgeons in Las Vegas. After the surgery, they determined that the mass in my left lung was cancerous. I followed all the necessary treatment and recovered once again. With all the trials and tribulations in my life, I think of all *God's* blessings bestowed on me. But in actuality, I know that my life is the result of following *God's plan* for me, and what's for me is for me! The *faith* I have in *God* to carry me through this life, as his plan is greater than any mountain of hopelessness. With the bad news finally behind us, I thought we were back in business again for good. I began to recover and realized that I was actually in retirement because of my illness and that I needed to go back to work until Barbara turned sixty-five.

In early 2004, I decided to go owner/operator again; this was always one of my endeavors as well. With the bad news finally behind us, we are back in business again. Using the Internet, Barbara and I found a tractor and trailer for sale in Denver, Colorado. We drove there in our van to make the purchase and loaded our van to the back of the trailer as we made our way back to Las Vegas. The tractor-trailer, with the van piggybacked on the trailer, is shown on the next page.

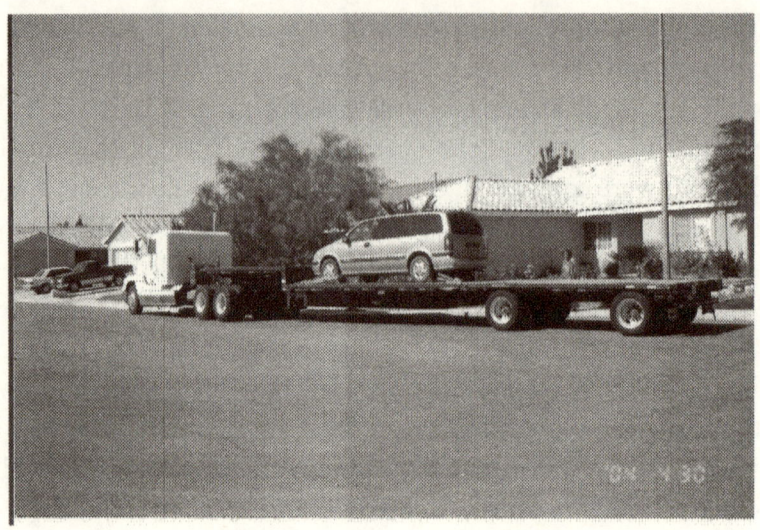

Van Piggy-backed On The Trailer

Barbara and I were hauling sheetrock from Las Vegas down to Phoenix. We would bring back materials to Home Depot or Lowe's, per our instructions. Barbara would travel with me, and this was good, because we worked at our own pace. However, in mid-summer of 2003, things took a turn for the worse. My father-in-law, Bill, had a stroke that rendered him bedridden; he also had one of his legs amputated. Cleo, Barbara's mother, had the burden of taking care of him at home. Cleo herself was not in good health; she was suffering with cancer too. As things got worse, Barbara being an only child felt compelled to leave North Las Vegas and go to Los Angeles to take care of her parents.

I decided to get other business contracts, closer to Barbara's family, that would take me to Southern California, so I could be close to the family. I started picking up materials from the Los Angeles Port and hauling from where the ships come in. I would pick up a load of materials from the ships that brought merchandise in from overseas. I would return to Las Vegas with a load and start all over again. The business was going well until I realized that my back was giving me so many problems. Many times, I had to park the tractor and trailer because pain made it hard for me to sit. This time, it was my back; I was in so much pain, I could barely climb in and out of the truck. I could not walk. But as always, I had *faith* that blessings would come and if it was *God's* will I would make it through this trial as well. Through all this pain and suffering, I kept my *faith* and continued to take one day at a time. In the meantime, my mother-in-law, Cleo, was taking care of Bill; Cleo lost her battle with cancer in September 2004. Cleo was loved dearly by Barbara and me. She was a kind and loving person who gave life her best efforts. We brought Barbara's dad, Bill, back to Las Vegas to live with us. By this time, I was very ill, and after facing back surgery in March of 2005, I was unable to walk without assistance.

After about a week of testing, I was referred to a rehabilitation facility and recuperation at Harmon Medical and Rehabilitation Hospital in Las Vegas. I slept in a hospital bed for two months, after which I had lost the ability to walk. The bathroom required constant upgrades and maintenance for convenience and safety. I was doing therapy every day. The Veterans Administration staff provided me with a walker with wheels and a seat so that I could stop and sit when I could go no further. Because of the pain and weakness I felt, I stopped frequently. Although my struggle for a healthy life continued into 2005, I was not going to be defeated and I knew it. After all I had been through with fighting this cancer, going through radiation treatment twice per day, finally my P.S.A level is 0.1. My last visit to my cancer blood specialist was January 20, 2006. I thank *God* I am living a normal life and working again with the ushers' ministry at Second Baptist Church. I am making a great effort to bring to the awareness of as many people as possible the thought, "what *faith* can do and what *faith* has done for me." Often, there were times I wondered if all the conditions, the illnesses I have suffered in life serve to keep me in place, in order with the Lord our *God*; I spend so much time on my knees. Now I will have to get up off my knees once again to face my destiny, but with the *faith* of a "mustard seed," I know *God* is not done with me yet.

Zucchini Plant "A Symbol of Faith"

As I sit on my patio in 2005, recuperating from my surgeries and looking at this zucchini plant that produced two squash, the first one harvested July 5, 2005, weighing ten pounds and measuring twenty inches long; the second weighing eight and three-quarter pounds, measuring seventeen inches long was harvested August 5, 2005; the third zucchini, weighing seven pounds, measuring sixteen and a half inches was harvested on October 31, 2005. Also, I observed that these two apple trees in my yard had a mass production of apples this year. I must remind you that we are living in a desert climate here in Las Vegas; today is the twenty-seventh of August and this plant still blooms in the midst of summer. The zucchini seed was planted in 2003, and nothing happened for two years, now this year 2005, its time has come. My wife Barbara and I kept eating the small zucchinis from the zucchini vine this year. Then one day, now 2005, *God* revealed to me that the one zucchini, closest to the ground, was larger and growing faster.

I got some wax paper from the kitchen, folded it up, and placed it underneath the zucchini, so it could slide more easily, and it did, allowing for growth movement. Then it was revealed to me; that's what my grandma Mandy's *faith* and prayers has done for me. Through my grandma Mandy's teaching and instilling the "faith of a mustard seed" and through her prayers, she put wax paper under my life so *God* could continue my growth movement through *faith*. It has never mattered about the tribulations I have faced; it has always been about the smooth surfaces made by Grandma Mandy's prayers on which I have been able to grow and expand. I still have my prostate, and thank *God* I can walk again, just in time to harvest perhaps one of the largest known zucchini ever grown in Nevada; a symbol of *faith*. I have spent thousands of dollars in radio, newspaper, and advertisements on this project, including my *www.letsgotoschool. com* Web site.

I made thousands of fliers, etc., trying to get some exposure. Finally, success, the zucchini turns out maybe to be one of the largest grown in Las Vegas Valley; I was blessed with the growth of this zucchini. I took it to the Spanish newspaper and they took a picture; this is what started the circulation of a zucchini as a symbol of *faith*. I give all praise and thanks to *God* for his wisdom, and my *faith* in "*his view of things*" continues to guide my *faith*. I think this story will demonstrate the value of *faith*, if it is in "*God's View*" of things. I have mailed flyers of the zucchini story to 200 churches in the Tulsa, Oklahoma area and 315 churches in the Los Angeles area, and many, many more to go.

Finally, I took the zucchini to the Channel 3 television station in downtown Las Vegas, where the weatherman for Channel 3 News was happy to show it on the weather report. This gave me great pleasure to be recognized for my *faith*. The Spanish newspaper *El Mundo* put it in their advertisement section on July 23, 2005; I passed out some zucchini flyers from the newspaper at Second Baptist Church during their usher meeting, where I am blessed to be a member of that board.

Traveling with the Zucchini

In 2005, Barbara, and I had decided to take a cruise. The third zucchini was ready for harvest, so I plucked it from the vine to take with us. My health had improved, and I felt at my best, now ready again to make a trip. Barbara and I had been planning a vacation for a while. During November, we packed our bags. I took flyers with me on vacation, and I held the zucchini in my arms like a baby, planning to take it everywhere. We headed for the Las Vegas Airport. We were on our way first to O'Hare International Airport in Chicago.

I gave out flyers to people; many of them asked questions about the zucchini as we continued on our way; some of the people asked me to sign the flyers. We went from Chicago to South Carolina, where we stayed with the Sampson family and visited the local library in Somerville, South Carolina. Also, I visited the Wesley Methodist Church. The people there were very curious about this large zucchini in my arms. From there in the South Carolina area, I left from Ladson, South Carolina and went on a cruise, on the Fantasy Cruise

Liner. While on the cruise, I took the zucchini to the Captain's Ball; it was quite a conversation piece.

After the cruise, we went on to New Smyrna Beach, Florida. While there, I stopped in the *News Journal* office on Canal Street with the zucchini. This news office editor wrote an article on the zucchini. Also, I have had articles written by the *El Mundo* Spanish newspaper and the *Las Vegas Sentinel Voice* in 2005. There is nothing greater than planting a seed, nurturing it as it grows, as *God* has planted me and guided my steps and now harvesting me, as I harvested the zucchini to wholesomeness. *Faith* has brought me to a preparation stage in my life, and *faith* shall continue to guide my future as trials and tribulations are only stepping stones on life's path.

Stepping Stones on Life's Path

I feel that my life has been shaped, because of *"God's Plan"* for the life of others who preceded me and the times I now live in. Some of those lives took on no noticeable path, yet others were shaped and placed in the spotlight by *God's* divine intervention. I know that I owe much gratitude to Dr. Martin Luther King, Jr., as all black Americans do, for paving the way to our future of non-violence in America. From this single act of courage and *faith*, the lives of others have been made free. I am thankful that *God* gave us Dr. King, for now my children and grandchildren have more opportunities to sit and study in an integrated classroom, to obtain the American Dream.

Like Dr. King had a dream, I too have a dream that this autobiography and memorials of my life will serve to support people who have fallen through the cracks in life, such as the homeless, children, and old folks who need early detection of cancer. I want to set the climate, where in Las Vegas and in every major city in America, we can address this issue with the intervention of big insurance companies dictating the treatment one can obtain. I was blessed to have adequate insurance to cover my expenses, through the years, and to be able share my blessings with those who are less fortunate. My dreams are to further develop the *www.letsgotoschool.*

com Web site to a point that it becomes a fully educational site for victims of cancer to read for *hope and education*. I pray for all cancer victims in this world.

I too am weary, like Rosa Parks, who refused to give up her seat in the colored section of a bus. Rosa Parks's single act of courage changed the momentum of the civil rights movement in America. She became known as the "Mother of the Civil Rights Movement." I am so thankful to reap the benefits of her action. Any American can now ride a bus and sit anywhere there is a seat, without worrying about the color of their skin.

I too hope that I have touched someone's life, as I have traveled through this world, and that I have achieved *God's Plan* for my life. I pray for the truck owners and truck drivers who deliver everything that we use, including the food on our tables. I pray for those driving the four-wheelers, praying they keep their cool on the road, avoiding road rage.

One day still, I want to record a song I wrote many years ago in 1992. The title of the song is "I Want to Walk Just Like Jesus Every Day." My dream is that at the end of my day, I want to speak to a large crowd of people with music playing in the background titled: "Sweet Hour of Prayer."

Celebration of Life:

On October 8, 2005, Barbara and I celebrated the lives of others with festivities in our home. We hosted a dinner for two truck-driving buddies who have been stricken with cancer. The dinner was served to over forty to fifty invited guests, with a menu that included: ham, beef brisket, barbecue ribs, hot links, turkey and dressing, black-eyed and rice, peas, mustard greens, potato salad, baked beans, dinner rolls, and cornbread.

The participating guests were blessed with our love of fellowship and it was our warmest wish to make all at home in our home. I played the piano as everyone sang the song "Jesus, Keep Me Near the Cross." Leading the chorus was my home boy and good friend. The food was blessed by a friend.

Cancer-Free

After blood work January 2, 2006, a chest scan January 9, 2006, and my visit with the cancer blood specialist January 20, 2006, I was pronounced *cancer-free*. *Thank God faith does work!* ***"I was knocked down, but got up again, and again, and again," I am still holding on to my ice cream.*** *God's Plan* is alive and working miracles through *faith* in my life!

Appendix

Appendix 1:Matt Davis's Genealogy

Matt's father and mother did not stay together long enough to raise Matt. Matt was raised by his grandma Mandy. Mandy was Matt's mother Rachel's mother. Matt's great-grandfather Jerry was Mandy's father; Great-Grandfather Jerry died when Matt was seven years old. He was eighty-four years old when he died. Matt is seventy-four years old now and he continues to give honor to *God* for blessing him and his wife Barbara, children, grandchildren, and other relatives. He has many grandchildren, including Evan, Gavin, Candace, Brittany, Shaunda, Brandon, Daniel, Teddy, Delesse, Celeste, Dana, Brice, and K.J. Prinston. Great-grandchildren are Shayla, Tyquon, Dimond, Desmond, and DeShawn. The Davis family has diminished. Matt has one sister left, Claritha, and one brother, Jesse Mack, and several aunts and cousins.

Matt and Barbara often took the two grandchildren Delesse and Celeste, who live with them here in Las Vegas. Their father assumed the care of these two grandchildren after their mother, Felicia was involved in a fatal automobile accident that occurred in Grambling, Louisiana on June 2, 2000, where they lived with the two children.

Appendix 2:   Matt in 1977 returns to the farm, using his knowledge of operating a tractor in the fields.

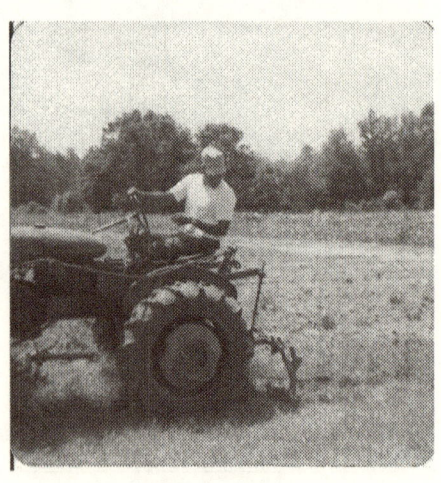

Appendix 3: Matt in 1977 on the farm, chopping weeds to allow the growth of good black-eyed pea plants.

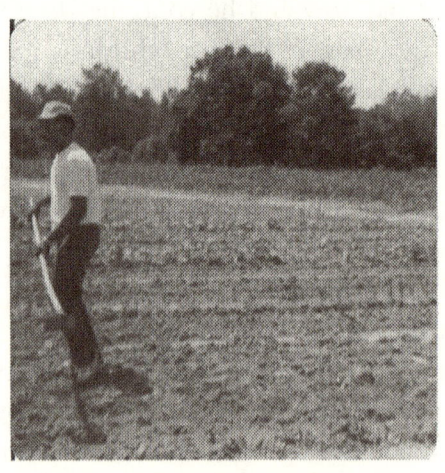

Appendix 4:Matt the Cancer Survivor: Man of Faith

Matt, *"The Miracle Man"* shown here after all his trials and tribulations with cancer:

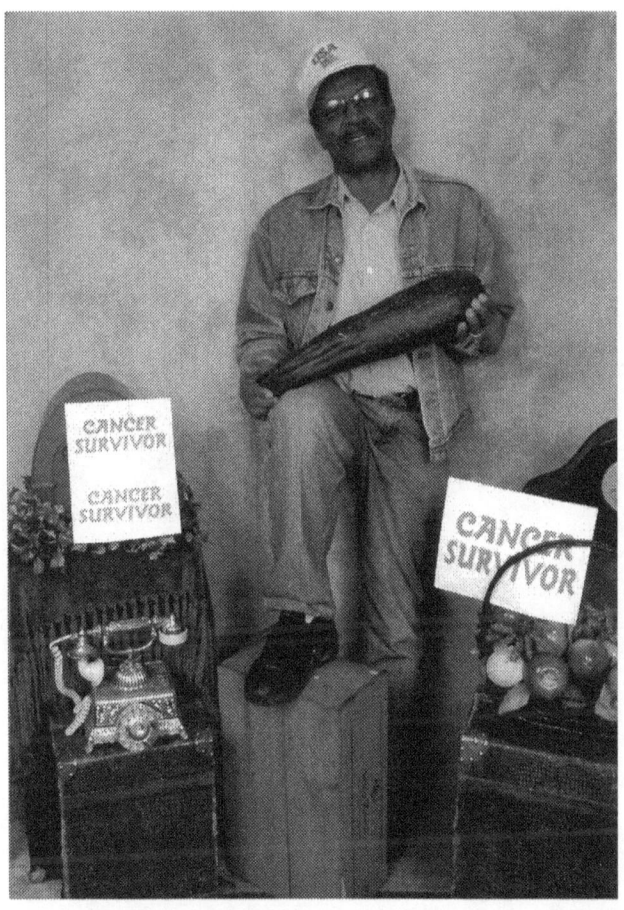

I plucked the third zucchini from the soil and took it with me everyplace and even on vacation in 2005, on a cruise. I took flyers with me on vacation, and I held the zucchini in my arms like a baby. Barbara and I headed for the Las Vegas Airport. We were on our way first to O'Hare International Airport in Chicago; from there on to South Carolina. In the South Carolina area, I left from Ladson, South Carolina and went on a cruise, on the Fantasy Cruise Liner.

While on the cruise, I took the zucchini with me for breakfast, lunch, and dinner, and even to the Captain's Ball; it was quite a conversation piece.

After the cruise, we went on to New Smyrna Beach, Florida. While there, I stopped in the *News Journal* office on Canal Street with the zucchini. This news office editor wrote an article on the zucchini.

Appendix 5: Matt's Mother, Rachel Rogers

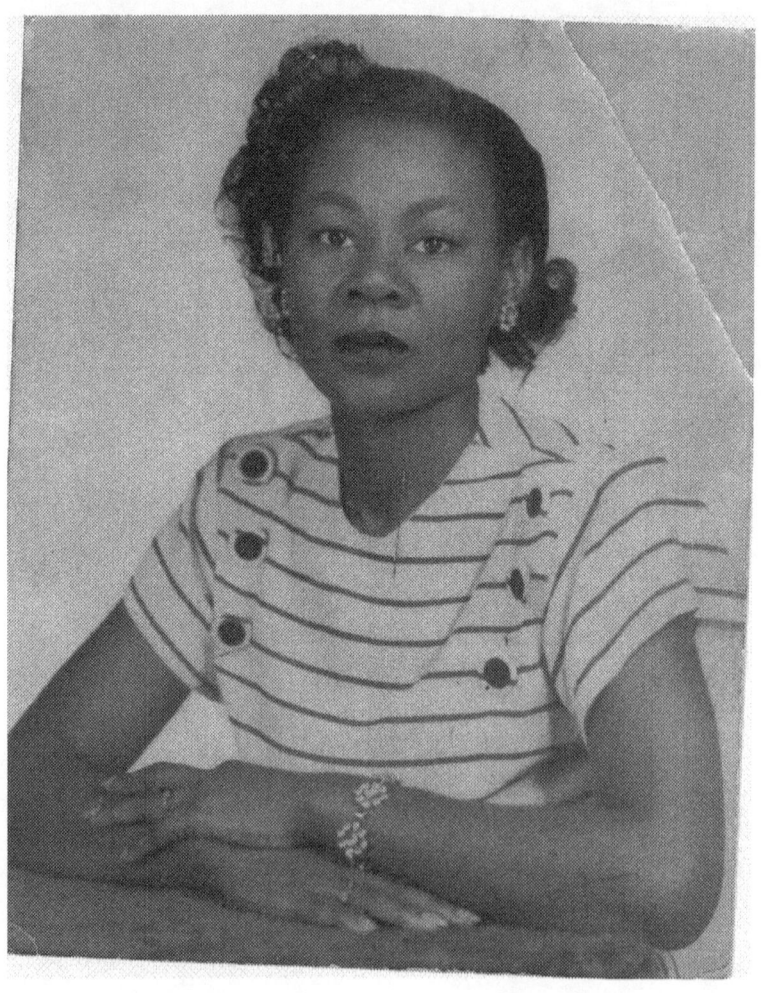

Appendix 6: Matt's Daughter

The first picture shown below is Matt's daughter, Deborah Lynn, former schoolteacher, now an insurance executive.

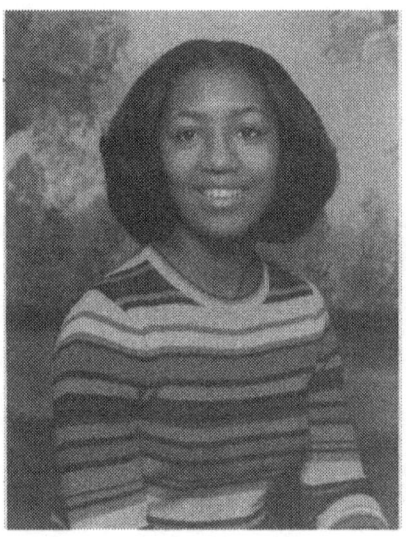

Appendix 7: Matt's Sons

Matt with his three sons: Terry Glen is an attorney in Montgomery, Alabama; sons Carl Matthews, Jr. and Kelvin Lewis both reside in Atlanta, Georgia. Carl Matthews, Jr., is a schoolteacher and playwright; Kelvin Lewis is a teacher and minister.

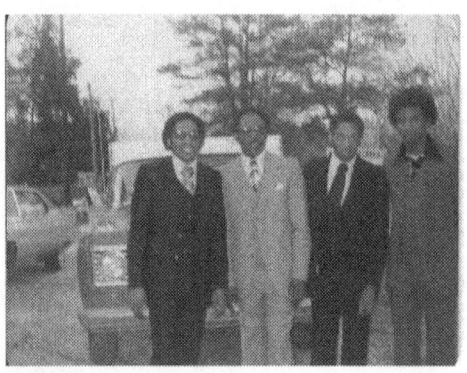

Appendix 8:Matt's Stepsons

Shown below are Matt's Stepsons Danny (left), Lynn (center), and Rodney (right):

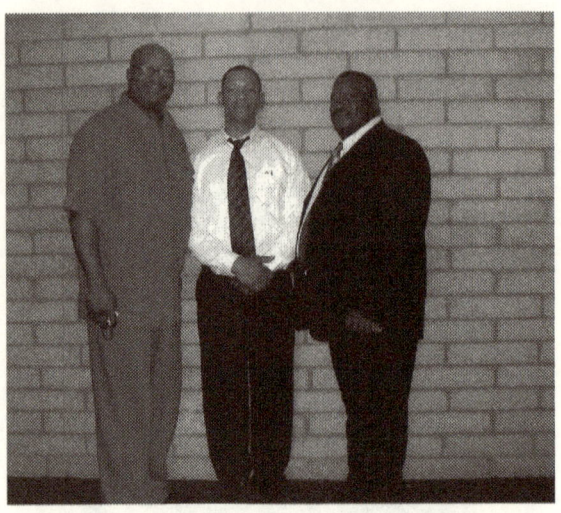

Appendix 9:   Matt's Place in Los Angeles, California.

Matt operated this business on Central Avenue at 18th Street in Los Angeles from 1974 to 1978.

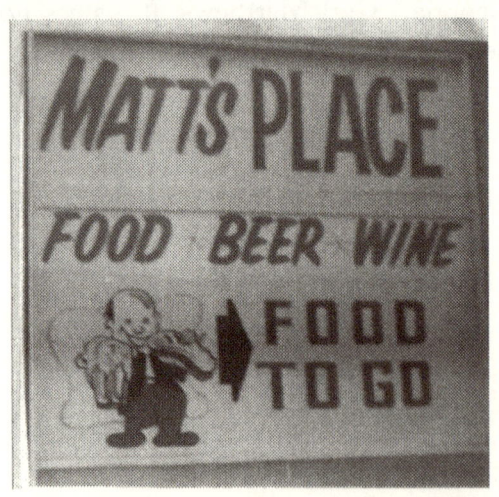

Appendix 10: Matt's Las Vegas Party Bus Services

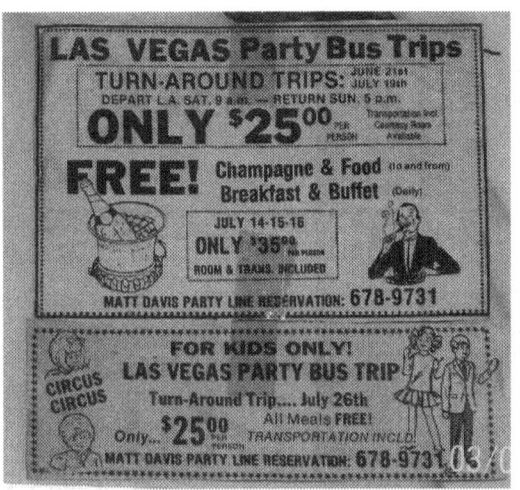

Appendix 11:Matt the Entrepreneur

Matt Davis as an entrepreneur is standing in front of one of his properties in Las Vegas, Nevada. He had no money, but was able to secure this property, as he would put it: *"I could not rub two quarters together of my own in 1986 when I purchased this building."*

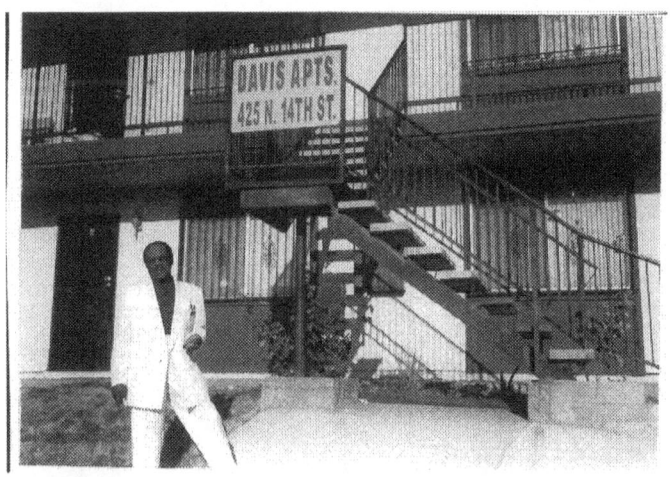

This apartment was a "four-plex," two bedrooms and one bath; equipped with stove, refrigerator, washer and dryer, and dishwasher. Barbara and I lived on the second floor, #D. I convinced the prior owner, Ray Chici, that I could pay the mortgage with no money down. The tenants were white families for many years because of the area in downtown Las Vegas. They were happy with my management, but had never had an African-American landlord before. The talk around the town was that Matt Davis was the first African-American landlord in downtown Las Vegas.

Appendix 12: Matt's Nevada Partners Certificate

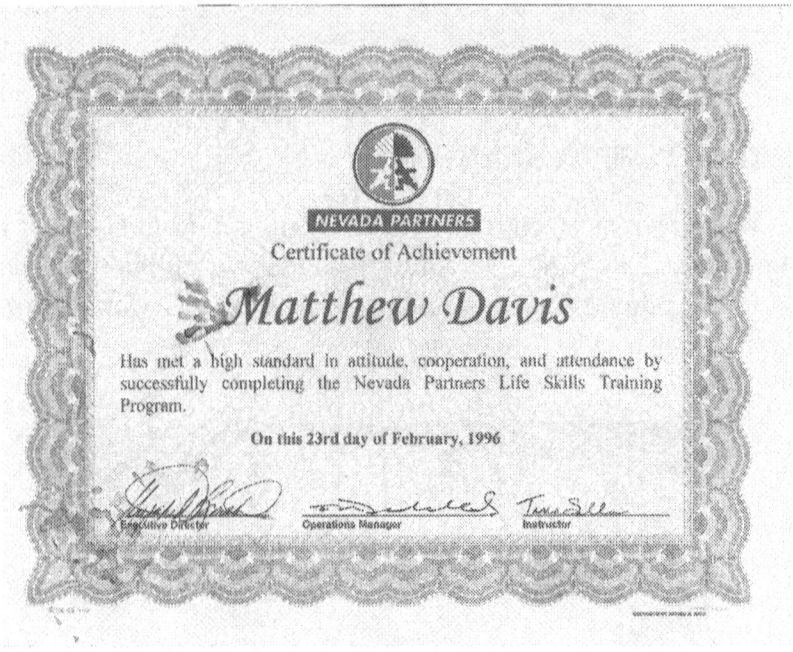

Appendix 13: The Entrepreneur and His "Let's Go to School" Logos - Grand opening of Let's Go to School Stationery, Inc., United States Patent and Trademark Office.

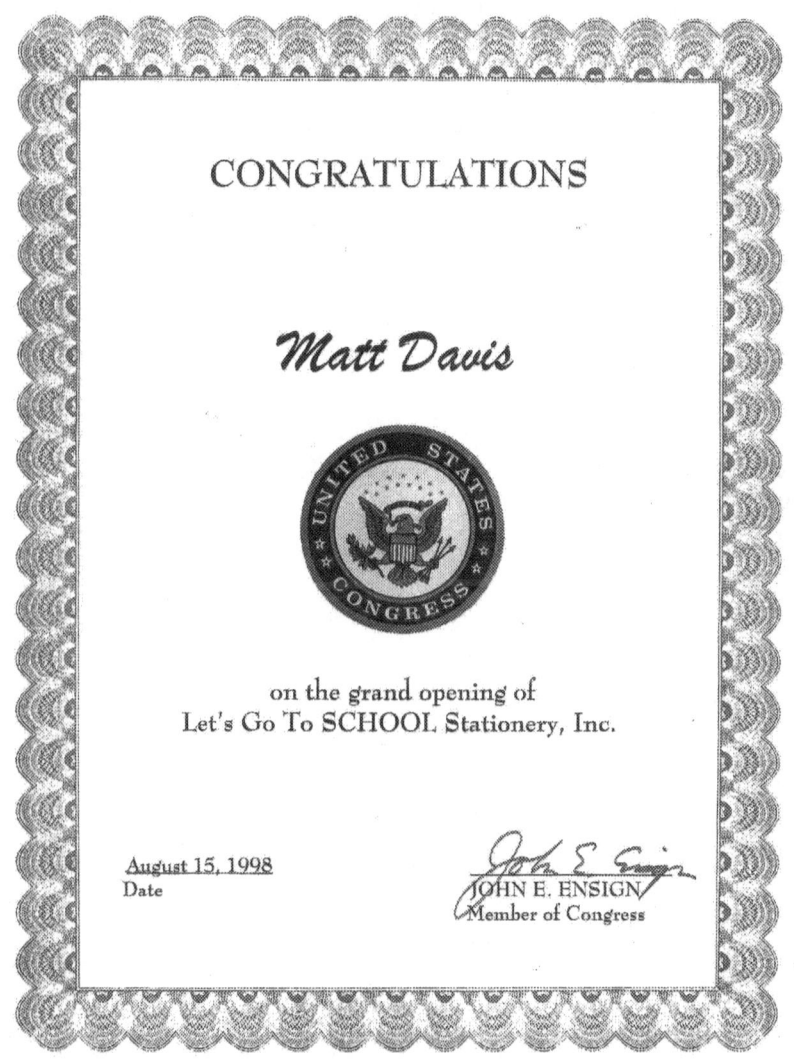

Grand Opening Of Let's Go To School Stationery, Inc.

Int. Cl: 16

Prior U.S. Cl.: 37

Reg. No. 1,721,093

United States Patent and Trademark Office   Registered Sep. 29, 1992

TRADEMARK
PRINCIPAL REGISTER

LET'S GO TO SCHOOL

FIRST USE   11-1-1990;   IN COMMERCE 11-1-1990
DAVIS, MATT (UNITED STATES CITIZEN)
618 EAST CARSON
SUITE 239
LAS VEGAS, NV 89101

SN 74-111,685, FILED 11-2-1990.

FOR:STATIONERY:NAMELY, NOTEBOOKS, NOTE CARDS,
WRITING PAPER AND EXAMINING
ENVELOPES, IN CLASS 16(U.S. CL. 37).
CORA ANN MOORHEAD, ATTORNEY

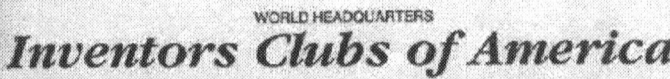

WORLD HEADQUARTERS

Inventors Clubs of America

A *Non-Profit* World Organization *to help* Inventors – Since 1935

October 11, 1990

Mr. Matt Davis
421 East Carson Suite 239
Las Vegas, Nevada 89101

Dear Mr. Davis:

It is my pleasure to inform you that at our
recent meeting of the Hall of Fame Awards
Committee, you were selected to receive the
NEW PRODUCT AWARD for your creative
letterheads and envelopes. Congratulations.

The awards banquet will be held on November
13, 1990 at the Radisson Hotel Atlanta
(downtown) at the corner of Courtland and
International Blvd. It will be necessary for
you to make your reservations prior to the
banquet as no tickets will be available at
the door.

We look forward to sharing this event with
you.

Sincerely,

Dr. Alexander T. Marinaccio
Chairman

ATM/gn

Inventors Clubs of America · Box 450261 · Atlanta, Georgia 30345 · (404) 938-5089

65

Appendix 13: Education Is the Key School Supply Truck

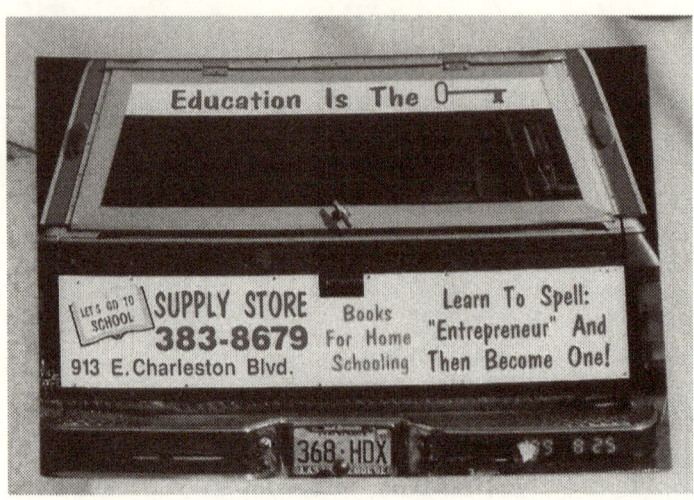

Appendix 13: Grand Opening of Store on
East Charleston Blvd., Las Vegas

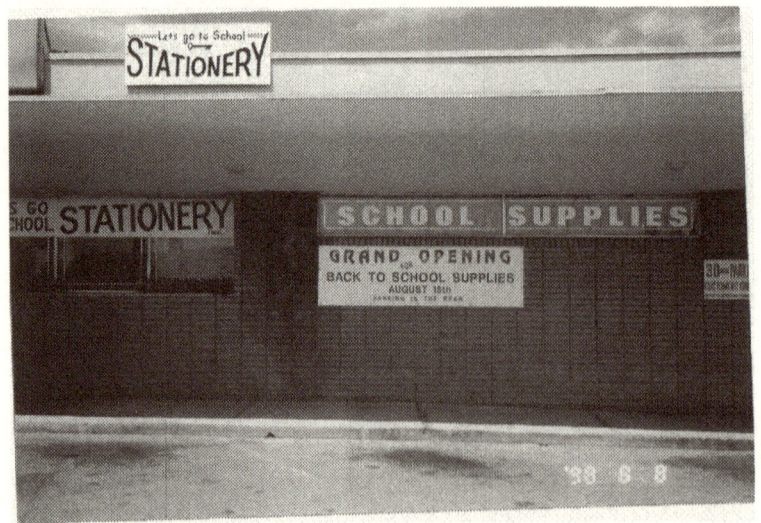

Appendix 13: Exhibit of School Supplies

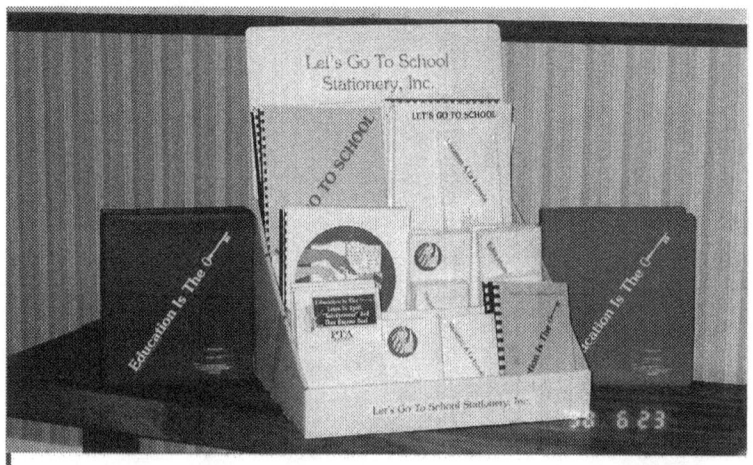

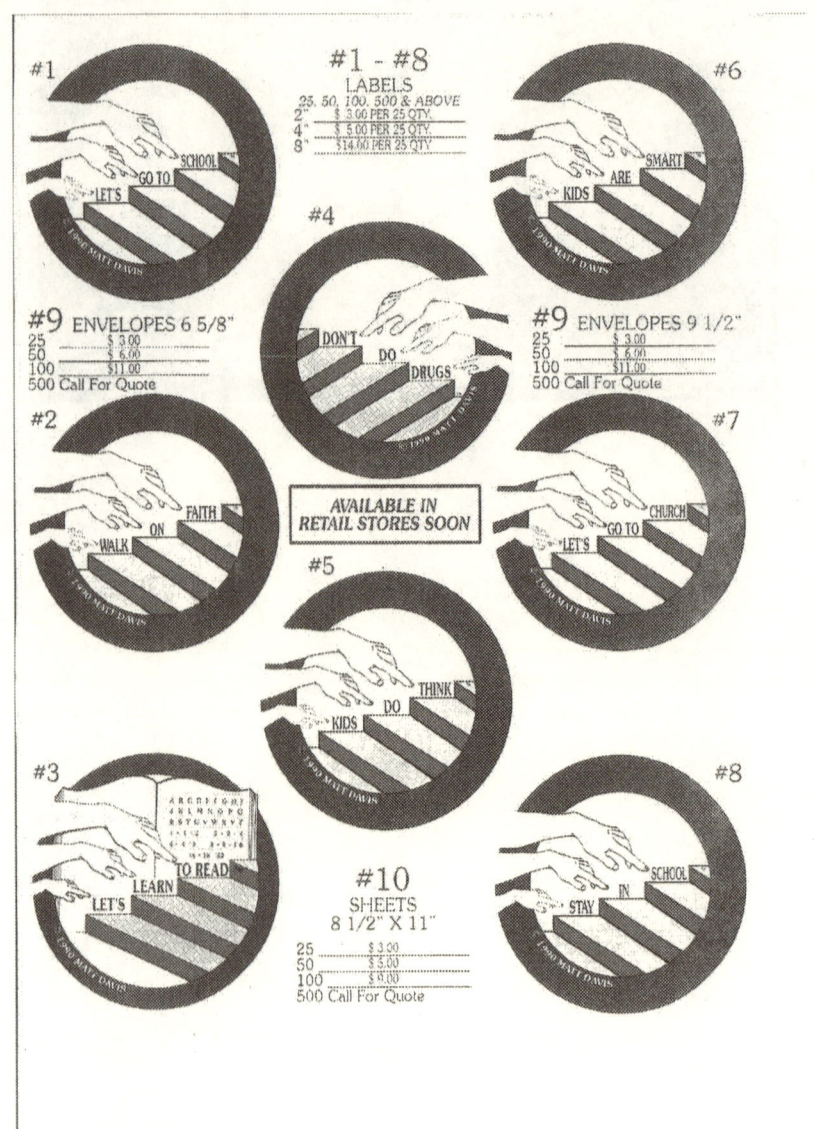

A B C D E F G H I*   1x1=1   2x2=4*
J K L M N O P Q R   3x3=9   4x4=16
S T U V W X Y Z   5x5=25

© 1995 Matt Davis. Let's Go To School Stationery

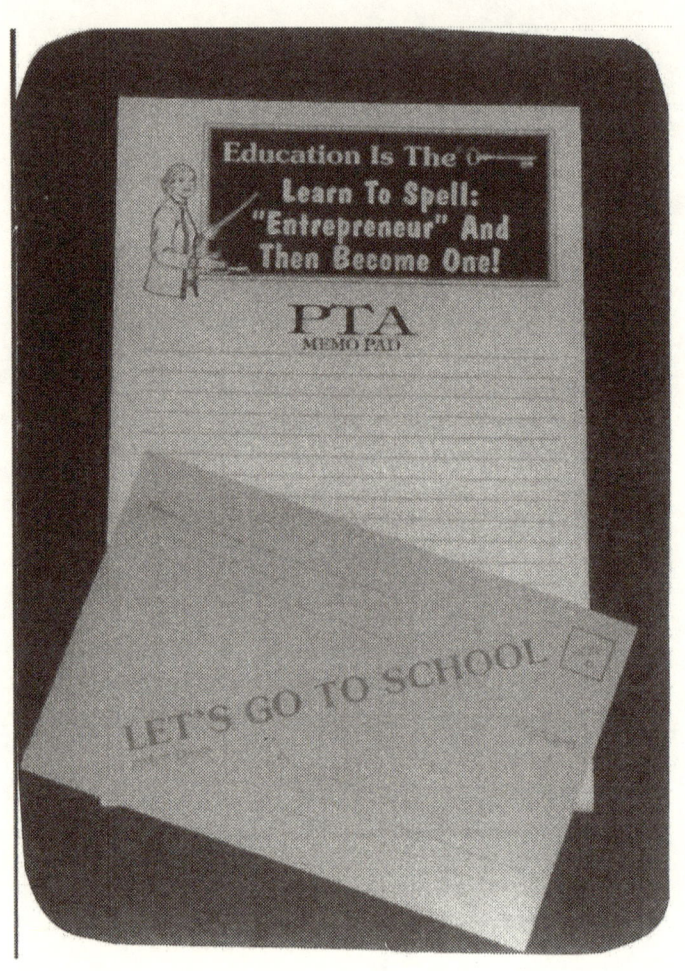

Appendix 13: Matt's "Poor Man's Copyright"

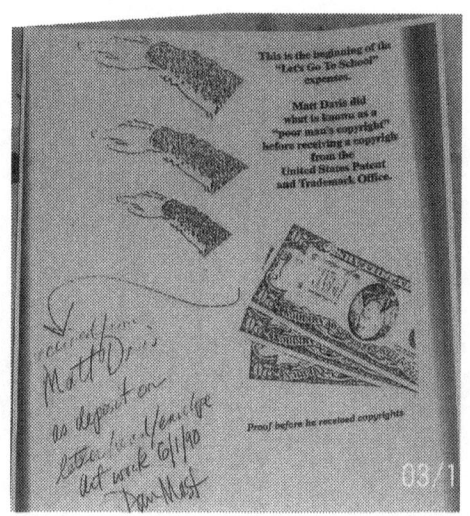

30,000 pieces of stationery were printed for Marines in Somalia as a donation.

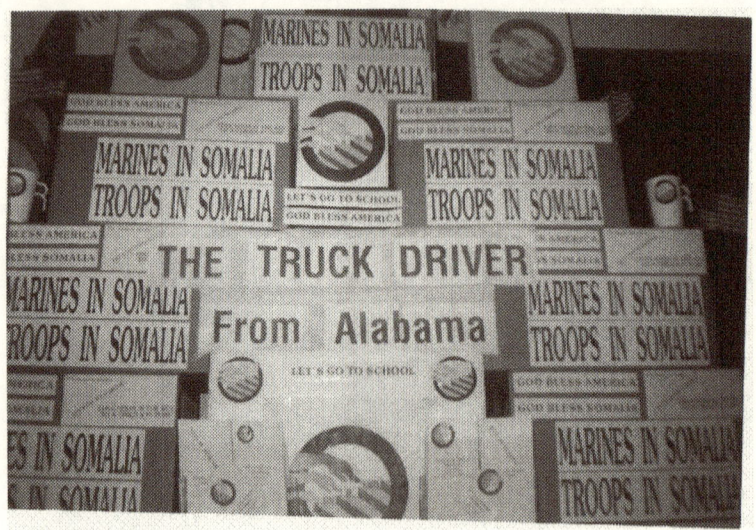

Appendix 13: Envelopes Supplies for Fundraiser in English

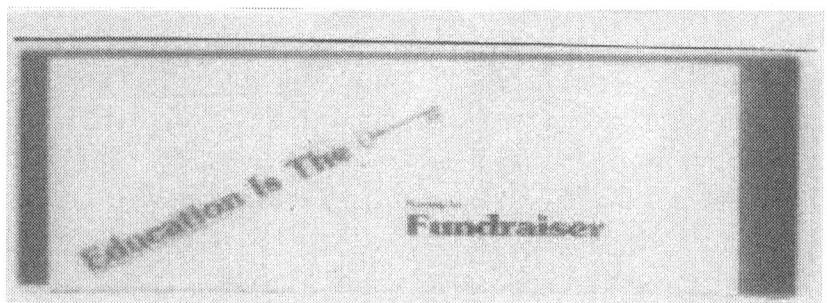

Appendix 13: Envelopes Supplies for Fundraiser in Spanish

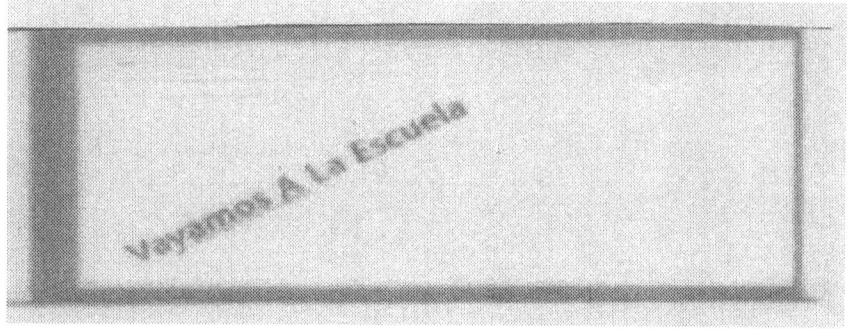

Appendix 14: Matt the Community Servant

Matt drove a Peterbilt Freightliner truck, as a community servant, in the Martin Luther King birthday celebration. The float was built by Matt, and in the designs of the float, he includes his "Let's Go to School" logos. The truck as a float is beautifully flocked with balloons and a picture of Martin Luther King. Matt Davis, the truck driver from Alabama, presents an educational episode of "Let's Go to School" and "Let's Learn to Read" in the Dr. Martin Luther King, Jr. Parade, January 19, 1991. Families were invited to see this educational event.

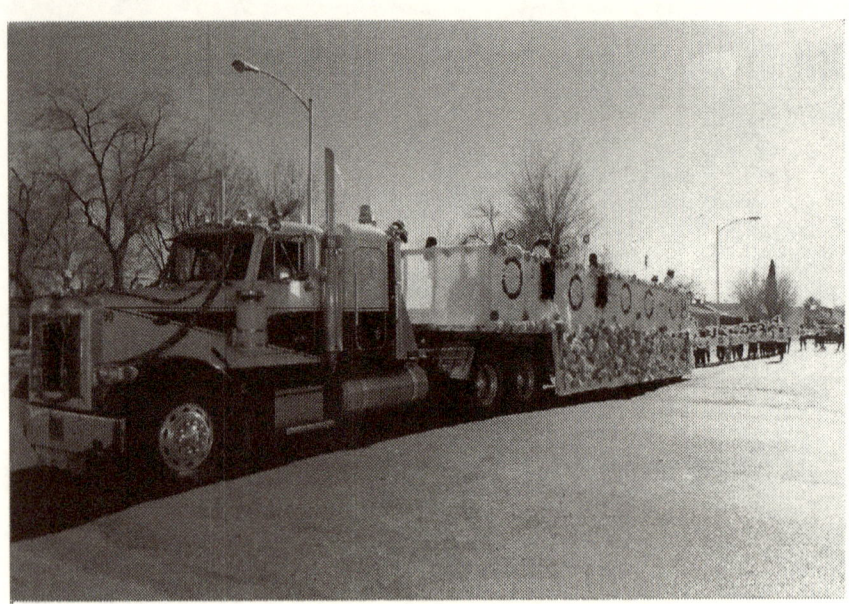

Appendix 15: Letter to America from the Truck Driver from Alabama

September 6, 1992

Mr. and Ms. Fellow Americans, Listen Up!

THIS IS THE TRUCK DRIVER FROM ALABAMA.

I have created a product for educational purposes as a business venture. This product will be implemented into the workforce and it will create many jobs for many people. It is not the total solution for this sagging economy, but it will sure put some meat and potatoes on many tables. It will create new ideas. It will create hope, and where there is hope, there is *faith*, and where there is *faith*, there is success, and where there is success, there is value.

So I say to all you folks, young and old alike, get your education now. I know that you are thinking that I just want to sell my product, and you are absolutely correct; but I also want to help stimulate this economy. We can do that by putting people to work. After the company has become a success, it will not only generate revenue for health insurance for the employees, but for our elderly people in this country who seem to have been forgotten. So I say to you, America, get your education now.

You see, I was born in rural Alabama during the Depression and I was raised by my grandmother, Mandy. Although she could neither read nor write, she taught me the value of *faith*. You see, I am not feeling sorry for myself because I am sixty-one-and-a-half years of age, and I plan to further my education once my LET'S GO TO SCHOOL product is on the market. I sincerely hope that many seniors will follow. Now, let me tell you about politics. You see, the conservative Republicans want everyone to be born rich, and that is not probable. And on the other hand, the Democrats want to use taxpayers' dollars on some programs that do not work because they do not follow through with the training and education for these people, which is so badly needed.

Now, listen to this — we have elected officials on both sides of which I have much respect for, and they are sitting there in Washington, DC with boxing gloves on and throwing rocks at each other and using large amounts of electricity. telephones, water, gas, wear and tear, and other utilities, not to mention time, when you should be gone fishing with your grandson or son, the best idea is to go shopping with your wife. I wrote President Bush a letter regarding this in January 1990. Now, you White House folks have had two hundred years to run this country correctly and you have failed consistently.

So, as I look back in remembrance of how Grandma brought us through the crisis, maybe it is time for us to start thinking about giving our women a chance to run this country. So, in essence, what I am saying to you Mr. Next President, if you fall short of correcting these many problems that our American people are faced with in this country, then sir, do not come back for seconds. And now the thing that I am going to say does not include females who are members of the departments.

Mr. Senate, Mr. Congress, Mr. House, all the above, you seem to forget our elderly people — the ones who made many roads possible for you to travel. And our worst-case scenario is not educating our young folks, who will be making your decisions in the future. So if you do not correct our major problems that we face today, y'all just line up and meet me behind Joe's place, leave your boxing gloves behind, but bring PLENTY OF TOOTHPICKS! My fellow Americans, ask not what education can do for you, but what you can do for education.

GOD BLESS AMERICA,
Matt Davis

Appendix 16: Politicians' Response to "Let's Go to School Logos"

Politicians and concerned influential citizens who responded to my letter campaign to solicit support for my "Let's Go to School" *logos program*:

11/27/91	Doug Wilder of Virginia
8/9/90	D.N.C. Ronald Brown
11/1/90	Donald Trump
2/29/92	John J. Johnson
6/18/90	Senator Edward Kennedy
6/26/90	Benjamin L. Hooks NAACP
9/11/90	Marilyn Quail
1/31/91	Oprah Winfrey
9/23/94	Oprah Winfrey
1/9/90	Boyd M. Tanner, Church of Jesus Christ of Latter Day Saints
7/17/91	Tom Mitchell, Las Vegas Review Journal
10/4/90	Ellen Chappell, C.B.N., Inc.
7/3/90	University of California
8/24/90	AARP
10/29/90	Nevada Governor Bob Miller
9/18/90	Congressman James H. Bilbray
7/31/90	Department of Education Maine
7/10/90	Department of Education South Dakota
7/19/90	California State Department of Education
7/18/90	New York State Education Department
7/5/90	Department of Education, State of Idaho
9/20/90	State of Ohio, Department of Education
2/5/91	Dunn & Bradstreet, Inc.
7/9/90	Texas Education Agency
4/10/90	Mississippi State Department of Education
5/11/92	President Bush
2/14/92	Community College of Southern Nevada
6/26/90	State of Oregon
6/30/91	US Department of Education, Washington, DC
7/18/91	Department of Education, South Carolina
7/5/90	Nebraska Department of Education
5/21/94	Hillary Clinton
9/18/95	Morgan State University, Baltimore, Maryland
7/31/91	Mayor Jan Lafferty Jones, Las Vegas Nevada
7/10/90	Commonwealth of Virginia, Department of Education
7/11/90	North Carolina Department of Public Instruction
11/20/90	Mead Corporation
10/26/93	Mead Corporation
6/6/92	Gibson Greetings
10/15/93	Gibson Greetings
3/10/92	Lamar Alexander

Appendix 17: Matt's letter to the president to abolish the word OLD, and other issues, written January 28, 1990.

This is a copy of the original letter that was sent, which reads as follows:

1-28-1990

Dear Mr. President:

This is an unusual request, but you are the big guy in this country, and I think you should be the first to know. I would like the word old abolished, when it is pertaining to a person after becoming fifty years of age. It could still be used when pertaining to material things and persons under fifty. I believe this idea will make many people happy to know that it's against the rules or just bad grammar to call them "old" anymore. I really would like to make it a misdemeanor, but we probably can't do that. This would give many people a great incentive, there will be less abuse, more respect, more love, less stress, longer life, just to name a few. We could replace that word with the word nice; of course, we will have to rewrite some books, but think of the number of happy people!

First, we need to know if the public wants this, if it can be done with minimum tax dollars. Just think, Mr. President, if we can get this over, you will no longer be an Old President, but a Nice one (smile). Mr. President, I am a registered Democrat, and I plan for my status to remain the same, but I have some ideas that will help you become the Education President that you promised to be.

Just one more request for now, Mr. President, that is for every registered voter to be given a card with numbers that can react into a computer system so the public can vote on some of the issues, especially some of the ones that Congress can't quite make up their minds on. There are many issues I think the public should have a voice in, even after voting our leaders into office. Maybe this can be done on a local or state level; if it works, and I am sure it will, then take it to the max.

I am sending a copy of this to my Senators and Congressmen and others.

Well, thank you for your time, Mr. President; maybe one day we can discuss these matters over a cup of coffee.

Thank you, Sir,

Matt Davis

The Truck Driver From Alabama
Matt Davis

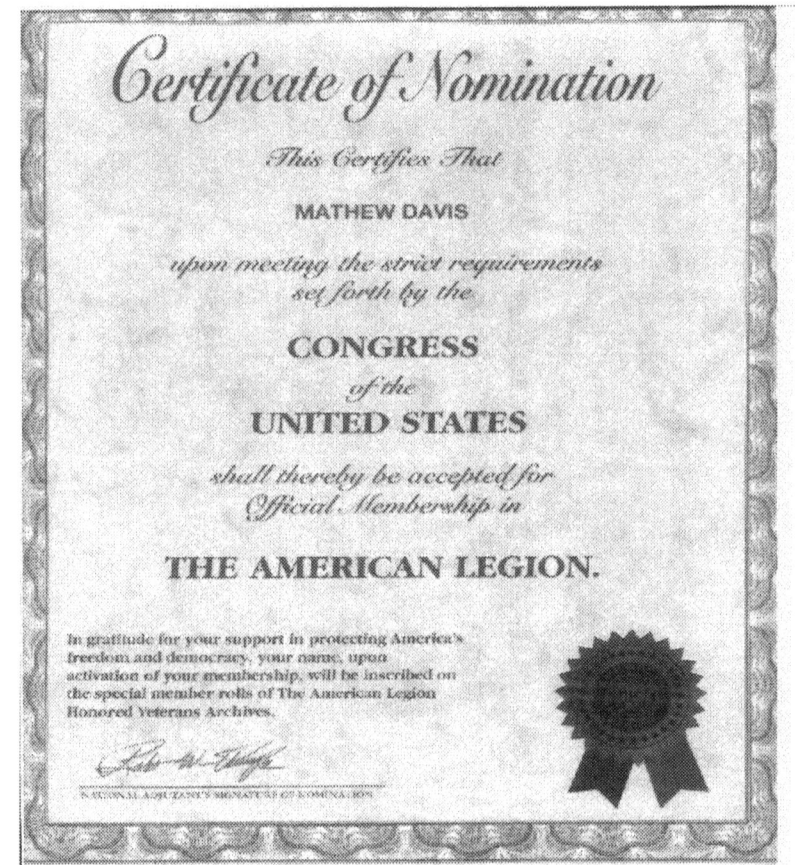

Appendix 19:   Matt's "Other Love"

Appendix 20:   Matt Davis, The Truck Driver from Alabama, Wrote:

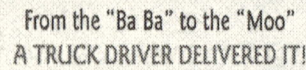

TRUCK DRIVERS' DELIGHT!

©**A proud truck driver from Alabama says:**® **Truck owners and truck drivers are special because everything you *see, feel, smell, use, drink, eat or hear* is delivered by truckers!**

From the "Ba Ba" to the "Moo"
A TRUCK DRIVER DELIVERED IT!

From the "Quack" to the "Crow"; the "Shrimp" to the "Alligator";

From the "Meow" to the "Bark" a truck driver delivered it! From the "Rooter" to the "Tooter" a truck driver delivered it!

Y'all Just Keep On Truckin'!

This article and much more are included in the soon to be published Autobiography by Matt Davis: The Truck Driver From Alabama.

Appendix 21:Community Achievement Awards

Celebrate Life 2003 from the Cancer Treatment Center of America, Trail Mixers – Vacation Bible School, New Product Award, "500 Men for Christ" from Second Baptist Church of Las Vegas, and Happy Father's Day Award from my children in 1998; and the Congress of the United States Official Membership in The American Legion.

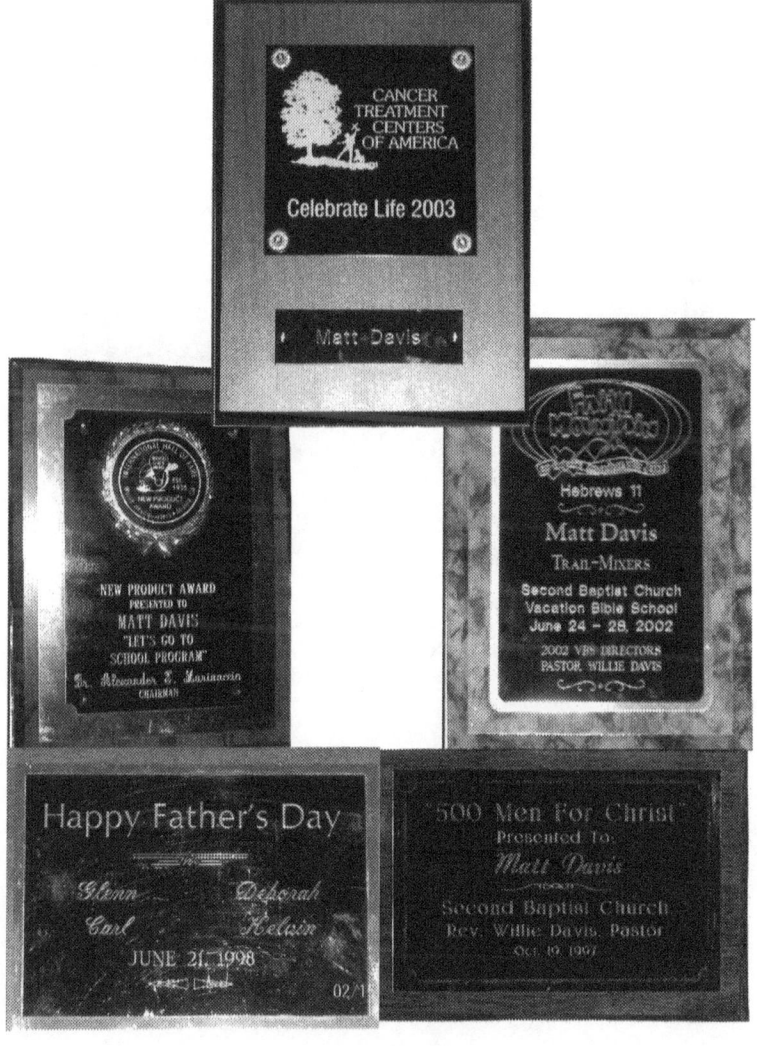

Appendix 22: Matt's Wife, Barbara J. Davis, paints a picture that marks the recovery of her husband.

This painting is of a road photographed in Wisconsin Dells in 2002. Matt is on the road to full recovery. Matt has cancer checkups every six months. He had blood work done on December 2, 2005; a chest CAT scan on December 9, 2005; and a visit with his cancer blood specialist on December 20, 2005, after which he was diagnosed as CANCER-FREE! Barbara painted this picture to signify that Matt is on the road to a healthy future once again! Matt envisions himself walking this road, as he sings his favorite song, "I'll Fly Away."

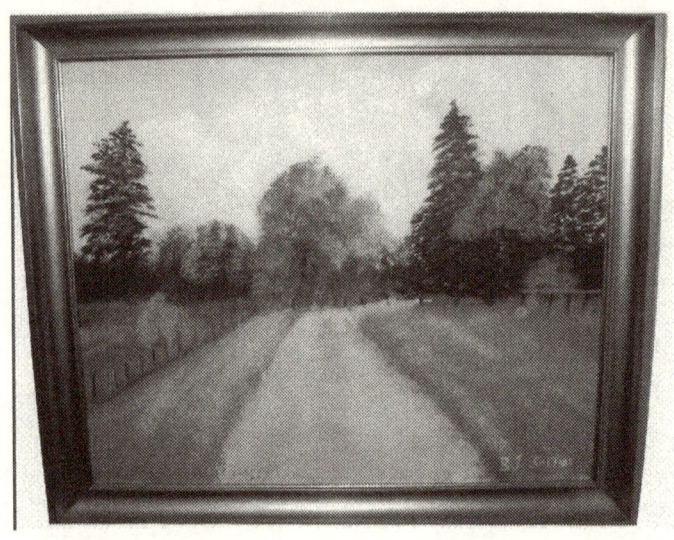

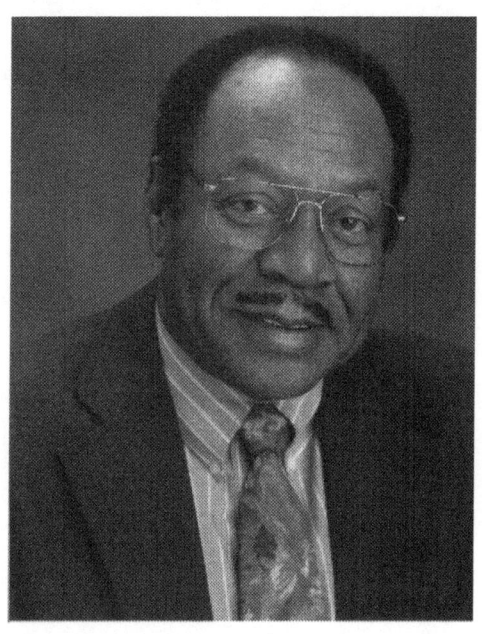

The Author

Matt Davis is a cancer survivor since 1995. He has overcome prostate cancer and lung cancer. In addition, he has had eye surgery to his left eye to reattach the retina, back surgery that left him unable to walk for a while; the cancer survivor is now seventy-four years young. The "Truck Driver from Alabama," believes that *faith* can do more than just move mountains!